The Roper-Logan-Tierney Model of Nursing

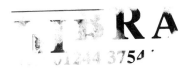
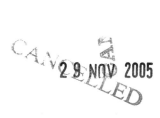

For Churchill Livingstone:

Senior Commissioning Editor: Jacqueline Curthoys
Project Manager: Gail Murray
Project Development Manager: Mairi McCubbin
Designer: George Ajayi

The Roper-Logan-Tierney Model of Nursing

Based on Activities of Living

Nancy Roper MPhil RGN RSCN RNT

Winifred W. Logan MA RGN RNT DSc(Hon)

Alison J. Tierney BSc(SocSc-Nurs) PhD RGN FRCN

Foreword by

Ann Marriner Tomey BS MS PhD FAAN
Professor of Nursing, Indiana State University, Terre Haute, USA

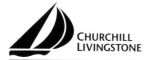
CHURCHILL
LIVINGSTONE

EDINBURGH LONDON NEW YORK PHILADELPHIA ST LOUIS SYDNEY TORONTO 2000

CHURCHILL LIVINGSTONE
An imprint of Harcourt Publishers Limited

First published 2001
Reprinted 2001

ISBN 0 443 06373 7

British Library Cataloguing in Publication Data
A catalogue record for this book is available from the British Library

Library of Congress Cataloging in Publication Data
A catalog record for this book is available from the Library of
Congress

Note
Medical knowledge is constantly changing. As new information
becomes available, changes in treatment, procedures, equipment and
the use of drugs become necessary. The authors and the publishers
have, as far as it is possible, taken care to ensure that the information
given in this text is accurate and up to date. However, readers are
strongly advised to confirm that the information, especially with
regard to drug usage, complies with the latest legislation and
standards of practice.

The
publisher's
policy is to use
**paper manufactured
from sustainable forests**

Printed in China

About the authors

Nancy Roper

Nancy Roper began her career as a full-time writer in the 1960s after 15 years as Principal Tutor in a school of nursing in England. Her first assignment on moving to Edinburgh and establishing her long link with Churchill Livingstone was as editor of *Churchill Livingstone's Nurses' Dictionary* and the *Churchill Livingstone Pocket Medical Dictionary*. Then followed her well-known textbooks *Man's Anatomy, Physiology, Health and Environment* and *Principles of Nursing*. Then,in the early 1970s, Nancy Roper studied for a MPhil degree at the University of Edinburgh and went on to become the first Nursing Research Officer at the Scottish Home and Health Department (1974–78) during which time she also carried out several WHO assignments for the European Office. It was Nancy Roper's MPhil research study, published in a monograph under the title of *Clinical Experience in Nurse Education* (1976), which provided the base for her later work with Win Logan and Alison Tierney. The first edition of their book, *The Elements of Nursing*, was published in 1980 and over the past 20 years Nancy Roper has undertaken speaking engagements in many parts of the world, talking with nurses and nurse teachers about the Roper-Logan-Tierney model.

Winifred Logan

On retiral from a distinguished nursing career, Winifred Logan was Head of the Department of Health and Nursing at Glasgow Caledonian University and previously was Executive Director of the International Council of Nurses (1978–80). She had already worked in North America and is a graduate of Columbia University, New York. Other international work includes serving as a WHO Consultant in Malaysia, Iraq and in Europe, and as first Director of Nursing Services in Abu Dhabi. Win Logan held a senior position in the Department of Nursing Studies at the Universityof Edinburgh for 12 years in the 1960s and 1970s before being appointed as Nurse Education Officer at the Scottish Office; and, at various times, she served on UK and international nursing and academic committees. Win Logan has honorary degrees from two universities and in 1996 was made an Honorary Fellow of the University of Edinburgh on the occasion of the 40th anniversary of the Department of Nursing Studies.

Alison Tierney

Alison Tierney was one of the first nurses in the UK to gain a PhD degree (1976) and to pursue a primarily research-orientated career. She was promoted in 1997 to a Personal Chair in NursingResearch at the University of Edinburgh, previously having been Director for a 10-year period (1984–94) of the internationally known Nursing Research Unit which was established by the Scottish Office in 1971 and based in the Department of Nursing Studies at the University of Edinburgh. Through her nursing and interdisciplinary research work and other activities, Alison Tierney continues to maintain close links with providers and users of nursing and health services. At national and international levels she has contributed to the strategic development of research in nursing through active membership of the Royal College of Nursing; as the RCN/UK representative on the Workgroup of European Nurse Researchers (WENR) during the 1980s; and as an Expert Research Advisor to ICN.

Contents

Foreword

Roper, Logan and Tierney collaborated to refine the Roper models and first published their thoughts in *The Elements of Nursing* in 1980 as a way of introducing beginning students to thinking about nursing practice. The five main interrelated concepts in their model are:

- Activities of Living
- Lifespan
- Dependence/independence continuum
- Factors influencing activities of living
- Individuality in living

At the time of the first edition (1980), death and dying, sociocultural factors and environmental issues were just beginning to be discussed, the inclusion of politicoeconomic factors was novel, and the topic of sexuality shocked some. The diagrams were redesigned for the second edition (1985), made to look less cluttered for the third edition (1990), and then left unchanged for the fourth edition (1996) with the exception of changing "physical" to 'biological'. This monograph (2000) is to be the authors' final publication and a lasting account of the model of nursing that has been the core of the Roper-Logan-Tierney publications since 1980.

The model is grounded in realism and accessibility. Roper-Logan-Tierney have taken the complexity of living and nursing and created a model that appears relatively simple, which is generally more difficult to achieve than a complex model. That simplicity allows the model to be readily understood, relevant and applicable to nursing practice; it provides a framework that helps learners develop a way of thinking about living and nursing in general terms; and it helps individualize nursing care. The model has been used in conjunction with the nursing process and medical practice. Because nursing care is not usually directly given by the registered nurse now, the model could be used for planning and to help teach families and aides how to individualize nursing care. It also helps shift the focus of nursing from ill-health to health, and facilitates health-promotion nursing practice and changes in personal lifestyle.Even though we want to emphasize wellness and independence now,people still do become unwell, become more dependent and need care.

Models are abstract systems of global concepts. They are not theory but they can help generate theory and organize thinking.The Roper-Logan-Tierney model was first developed when there was almost no published literature about nursing theory, before the seminal Fawcett (1984) and Meleis (1985) books. The authors had familiarized themselves with the early North American work of Henderson, Orem, Rogers, and Roy even though that literature was rare in UK nursing libraries.

The Roper-Logan-Tierney model has been widely used in Europe and has been translated from English into eight other languages: Dutch, Estonian, Finnish, German, Italian, Lithuanian, Portuguese and Spanish. In addition, the model has been used in Africa, Australia, India, the Far East and South America. It has been taught widely in UK colleges of nursing, and it is a popular choice when a model is used in practice in the United Kingdom. Although this monograph presents the authors' final account of the Roper-Logan-Tierney model, it need not be the final version.The authors now leave it up to others to test the concepts and refine the model.

Ann Marriner Tomey

Preface

In the preface to the last edition of our well-known textbook *The Elements of Nursing* (fourth edition, 1996), we noted our reservations about perpetuating the publication of a book beyond its useful life. In place of any further editions of *The Elements of Nursing* we decided to prepare a final publication—this monograph—in order to provide a lasting account of the *Model of Nursing* that has been at the core of all Roper-Logan-Tierney publications ever since it was presented in the first edition of *The Elements of Nursing*, published in 1980.

Our reasons for getting together in the mid-1970s to develop our Model of Nursing, which is based on a Model of Living, are explained in Chapter 1. This opening chapter is intended to provide readers with some understanding of the background to our work, including the circumstances prevailing in the nursing profession and the wider healthcare context at that time. Over time, as documented in each of the four editions of *The Elements of Nursing*, we have continued to refine the model, and the latest account of the model—our last—is now to be found in this monograph.

The model of living, which is centred on Activities of Living, is described in Chapter 2, and in Chapter 3 the model of nursing is presented. Unlike *The Elements of Nursing*, this publication concentrates only on the model and its component concepts. There is no attempt to include the many examples of application of the model in the process of nursing (i.e., assessing, planning, implementing, evaluating) which, all with supporting references, made up a major part of each of the four editions of *The Elements of Nursing*. The application of our model is now left to its users and, as we have emphasized repeatedly, we would not want this model, or any model, to be 'set in stone' and so we hope that there will continue to be creative use and further development of our model in the future.

The controversial question of whether nursing models in general, and the Roper-Logan-Tierney model in particular, do have a continuing role in twenty-first century nursing is debated in Chapter 4, the closing chapter of this monograph. This chapter is based on a paper that was presented at the First International Nursing Theory Conference held in Germany in 1997. The arguments for and against nursing models are examined and the chapter provides a critical self-assessment of our own model. The intention is to encourage the continuation of critical—but informed—debate about the role of models and conceptual thinking in nursing.

Our own thinking about nursing has been shaped and challenged by those nurses, teachers, students and scholars who, over the years—and from around the world—have shared with us their interpretation, use and criticism of our model. We acknowledge with thanks their contributions because they have enriched our discussions, provided encouragement and given direction to our ongoing refinement of the model.

We are delighted that our final Roper-Logan-Tierney publication comes with a foreword written by Professor Ann Marriner Tomey, originator of the internationally known book *Nursing Theorists and Their Work*. Ann's interest in our work has been much appreciated and, in the fourth edition of her book (which is co-edited with Martha Alligood and was published in 1998), a chapter is included on the Roper-Logan-Tierney model of nursing. Importantly, that publication has extended access to our model, particularly for North American nurses, and we hope that *this* publication will ensure that there is lasting access to the Roper-Logan-Tierney model when *The Elements of Nursing* is no longer in print.

Nancy Roper
Win Logan
Alison J. Tierney

Edinburgh 2000

1

Introduction

This monograph describes the Roper-Logan-Tierney model of nursing which was first published in *The Elements of Nursing* in 1980. It was an attempt to present nursing students with a conceptual framework identifying the theoretical base that underpins nursing practice across healthcare settings. In subsequent editions of that textbook (1985, 1990, 1996) our ongoing refinement of the model was explained in the text and, for the purposes of this publication, the various revisions of the model are summarized in Appendix 1.

The Roper-Logan-Tierney model was not created, primarily, as a contribution to the theoretical literature; it was essentially for educational purposes—for beginning nursing students and their teachers. However, practising nurses also showed interest, and the Roper-Logan-Tierney model of nursing was the first UK model to be used extensively in a variety of practice settings. Indeed, it is now known in many parts of the world (*The Elements of Nursing* has been translated into eight other languages) and it has been one of the prescribed introductory textbooks for nursing students in many schools of nursing since its initial publication in 1980. While the detail of the textbook has needed to be extensively updated with each new edition, the *model* on which it is based has remained relatively intact although, as noted, there have been several refinements since 1980. Therefore, rather than prepare a fifth edition of *The Elements of Nursing*, this monograph provides a more lasting account of the *model* itself. It is left to the user of the model to translate the concepts into practical applications that suit local circumstances or that relate to the needs of nursing students at different stages of their education.

Before describing the model, it is interesting to put it in context by attempting to take a global view of prevailing conditions in nursing, and in healthcare provision, during the period from the 1950s to the 1970s which preceded—and prompted—the original development of the Roper-Logan-Tierney model. First, a brief résumé of the development of conceptual models of nursing, in general, is provided.

Conceptual models of nursing

Attempting to describe nursing is not new. *Notes on Nursing; what it is and what it is not* is the title of the book written by Florence Nightingale in 1859. Although written in the nineteenth century, some of her views are peculiarly apt in today's world. For example, Nightingale maintained that the 'laws of health' and the 'laws of nursing' are in reality the same, and she placed great emphasis on the relationship between health and the environment. However, identifying the knowledge required as a basis for nursing practice, and indicating how the many disparate types of knowledge are interrelated and combined to provide a coherent framework for nursing—a conceptual model—is a twentieth century development.

The idea of using conceptual models in the context of nursing had its origin in North America. Perhaps North American nurses were in the vanguard because educational preparation of nurses began to be centred on universities 50 years before that opportunity was provided in the UK—indeed, in Europe. In the USA, the first nursing programme for beginning students that was university based dates from 1907 at the University of Minnesota, whereas the first in Europe was not established until 1960 at the University of Edinburgh, Scotland.

In the academic setting of a university, scholarship and research are an expectation. By the early 1950s, a number of American nurse scholars including Peplau (1952) and Henderson (1955) were publishing their personal views about the nature of nursing: in fact, Henderson's ideas quickly became known worldwide when she was asked by the International Council of Nurses to prepare the booklet *The Basic Principles of Nursing Care* (1960), which is now available in almost every language. At the time, however, these writers did not use the term 'model of nursing'.

Meantime, nurse education in American universities had to produce curricula acceptable to both academia and to the nursing profession, curricula that would exhibit a meaningful framework and give coherence to the different subjects studied by beginning students. Delineation of a body of nursing knowledge was necessary.

By the 1960s and early 1970s, a number of North American nurses, using data and experience collated during years of participation in nursing research, nursing practice and nursing education, were developing personal perspectives on the nature of nursing. They began to refer to their image of nursing as a 'conceptual framework' or 'model' (e.g. Orem (1959), Johnson (1959), King (1964), Levine (1966), Rogers (1970), Roy (1970) and Neuman (1972)), and later they added refinements to their early work. The historical evolution of models of nursing is described in detail by Meleis (1997) in *Theoretical Nursing: Development and Progress*, and analyses and evaluations of different models have been published, for example by Fawcett (1995), Marriner Tomey & Alligood (1998), and Aggleton & Chalmers (2000). These recent publications contain many references to articles and books written by the above-named model-builders, making it possible to chart the ongoing refinements in the thinking of each model-builder over a period of time. Scrutinization of their original work gives a better appreciation of the full significance of their individual contribution to nursing knowledge.

Theorizing about nursing is fascinating and academically challenging, but if a model is to be useful for the practice of nursing there must be a vehicle for translating the model into a usable form. The introduction of the 'nursing process' provided a means for this 'translation' of nursing models into practice. This process, this logical mode of thinking—assessing, planning, implementing, evaluating—is used in many disciplines: it is not peculiar to nursing, and this cyclical process was advocated as a way of operationalizing the concepts used in the nursing models.

This was the stage of development in the 1970s when the literature about models of nursing and about the nursing process was beginning to be discussed more widely in the UK; and there certainly were a number of nurses who treated such ideas with derision, and dismissed them as 'armchair theorizing' from across the

Atlantic which would not work in the UK. So what were the trends in the nursing profession and in nursing practice that led to the circumstances prevailing in the 1970s, and which prompted this interest (and disinterest) in nursing models?

Trends in nursing in the UK: 1950s to 1970s

Perhaps some of the criticism exemplified by the 'it wouldn't work in the UK' argument was justified. After all, those models produced by the North American nurses focused on the importance of the individual client/patient. Admittedly, in the UK, in the 1950s and the 1960s, most nursing was not planned around the consideration of clients/patients as individuals. In most hospitals nursing was still *task orientated* and there was no recorded assessment and comprehensive plan for the nursing of each individual patient.

Even so, there were many excellent nurses who provided effective, compassionate care. These 'good' nurses were, in effect, using a mode of thinking akin to the nursing process but they did not analyse or explicate what they were thinking or doing in terms of a process or steps within it; nor did they document information related to each patient in an ordered or comprehensive manner; and, importantly, the outcomes of the patient's nursing care were not evaluated systematically. Because nurses did not explain or record nursing, there was no tangible evidence of the *intellectual* aspect of the process to the onlooker, who saw only the observable behaviour of the nurse. Thus, for the onlooking nurse learner in particular, it was difficult to appreciate and understand the often rapidly executed mental activity that determined the experienced nurse's actions. So the results of the 'good' nurse's thinking were neither evident nor systematically evaluated.

This was not surprising. In the 1950s, the nationally prescribed curriculum for general nurses stipulated that during studentship most of the practice placements were in hospital settings (i.e. disease settings). In fact, student nurses were virtually inexpensive 'pairs of hands' to staff the hospitals. This hospital orientation and medical model of health care were reflected in the educational programmes. Doctors provided a considerable proportion of the lectures in schools of nursing and, inevitably, these were based on disease conditions and centred on medical treatments. Although there were exceptions, most nurse teachers did not provide any organized substantial back-up which showed the relationship of disease conditions to the patient's psychological or social or cultural or economic circumstances, and how, together, they might influence the patient's response and nursing interventions. In summary, the preparation of student nurses was task orientated, disease orientated, biologically orientated and hospital orientated, and there was little progress towards identifying an organized body of nursing knowledge.

However, a sizeable number of nurse leaders in the UK were increasingly aware that the knowledge base of nursing must be explicated; that the individuality of the client/patient must be recognized as the focus of nursing; that health and the prevention of disease should be given more emphasis; and that relevant changes must be made in the educational programme for beginning nursing students. Increasingly, nurse practitioners and nurse educators spoke out about the need for change and publicized their ideas in the nursing literature. Over the years, too, various reports commissioned by the government and by the profession itself advocated that students should cease to be the mainstay 'pairs of hands' in hospitals; that, although experience in practice areas was essential, educational objectives should be paramount during nurse studentship; and that the entire system of basic nurse education should be reorganized to provide a theoretical base in settings which were health orientated as well as disease orientated.

Gradually, in hospitals, different methods of organizing nursing were introduced such as patient allocation, team nursing and primary nursing, and with these changes came a gradual shift away from task orientation to patient orientation. Eventually, the content of the basic nursing programme was altered to include, for example, experience in a psychiatric setting in which the importance of psychological aspects of nursing were, at least, introduced; and experience in a community setting where the student had an opportunity to become acquainted with the significance of some of the social, economic and environmental issues that might influence a client's health and lifestyle.

Over time, various experimental programmes emphasizing some of these changes were implemented and evaluated, and eventually some programmes were established in a university setting, the first in the UK being at the University of Edinburgh in 1960. It was in the context of these nursing developments in the

UK that the Roper-Logan-Tierney model of nursing was conceived and formulated in the mid-1970s.

Of course, nursing and nursing models cannot be considered in isolation. Nursing is part of a healthcare system within the broad framework of the society it serves. The changes that had been taking place in nursing during the middle decades of the twentieth century were, in part at least, a reflection of changes that were occurring in healthcare systems at large.

Trends in health care in the UK: 1950s to 1970s

It is interesting to reflect on the prevailing conditions in the UK when the National Health Service (NHS) was introduced in 1948 immediately after the Second World War. The provision of a national healthcare system, free of charge at the point of need, was a prodigious innovation which undoubtedly has influenced a number of improvements in the health of the nation and has inspired the development of health services in other parts of the world.

In hindsight it sounds naive, but in the immediate post-war years the idea still persisted that there was a 'hard-core' of ill-health in the nation that could be 'removed' by providing a free health service; in fact, it was believed that as people's health improved the overall costs to the government would be reduced. On the contrary, the costs of health care were destined to soar. In the post-war period in the UK, there were nationwide changes in the social, economic and political circumstances, and inevitably these influenced the direction of growth in the fledgling NHS. Many merit mention but two had a direct impact on the development of costly hospital provision, not only in the UK but in most of the Western world.

The first was the growing challenge to health services arising from changing demography, particularly the increasing number of elderly people, and the proportion of the population aged over 65 years. The phenomenon of population ageing arose from the convergence of two trends: the long-term downward trend in the birth rate creating an increasingly large proportion of older people in the population; and the trend of increasing life expectancy (in the UK in 1901 it was around 52 years, in 1951 around 66 years, and by the beginning of the 1990s it was 72 years for men and 78 years for women). There were, and still are, many healthy elderly people in the population but, inevitably, the greater incidence of disease in this age group gradually began to make greater demands on health services in general, and on hospital services in particular.

The second development contributing to rising healthcare costs was the increasing use in health service facilities of the knowledge available from technological advances, which began to accelerate in the second half of the twentieth century. More sophisticated and more effective treatments became available for a number of disease syndromes; popular demand for access to 'cures' of more and more esoteric disorders increased; expensive hospital specialties were established to meet the demand (they were labour intensive and resource intensive); the use of new costly drugs proliferated; and the overall expense of the NHS soared out of all proportion to original estimates. So, even by the 1970s, in terms of allocation of finance (and this concern increased in the 1980s and 1990s) and, indeed, focus of attention, the NHS seemed hospital orientated, disease orientated and medically orientated. In fact, extremist critics maintained it was a misnomer to refer to a health service: it was a 'sickness service'.

But that was not the whole picture. Health-orientated services were also available and, within these services, nursing was making a valuable contribution, for example in maternity nursing, health visiting, school nursing and occupational health nursing. Even while hospital provision was becoming so dominant, there was increasing interest, in some quarters, in the services that actively promoted health, maintained health and prevented disease. It was recognized, however, that, in terms of the public's perception, the results of these types of activities were not so dramatic as the results of disease intervention; and health professionals were aware that the outcomes were more subtle to identify, more difficult to measure, and more elusive when attempting evaluation of outcomes—and therefore more difficult to justify for financial resourcing.

By the 1960s and 1970s, too, improved educational provision meant that the general public was better educated and also better informed about, for example, health and illness, partly because of the increasing sophistication and effectiveness of the mass media. In contradistinction to a 'nanny-state' mentality which was initially engendered in response to providing health services free of charge, the idea was propagated that, although the government made considerable provision, individuals also had some personal responsibility for their own state of health, and for the lifestyle they adopted for themselves and their families. Similar developments were occurring in other developed countries, many of which had adopted a form of government-funded or government-led health service in the wake of the Second World War.

These various trends in the approach to health and disease were debated at an international level in 1978 at the World Health Organization–United Nations Children's Fund (WHO/UNICEF) conference in Alma-Ata in the former USSR, which involved both developing and developed countries. The recommendations arising from the discussions spelled out an ambitious blueprint: 'Health for all by the Year 2000'. Health, it was emphasized, was not merely the absence of disease but the opportunity to create well-being and to maximize human potential. Hospital services were still part of the 'H2000' plan but the need for community services was highlighted; the provision of care in the home setting was commended; and the promotion of health and prevention of disease were stressed. Political will was needed at national level involving governmental agencies that determined the social, economic and environmental conditions conducive to healthy living. Nevertheless the people themselves must accept some responsibility at a local level. Personal behaviour, and its influence on living conditions, was a significant factor in promoting health and well-being. The UK was one of the 134 countries represented at the WHO/UNICEF conference and subscribed to the general principles of the H2000 recommendations.

Although this is admittedly a much abridged and selective view of events during the 1950s to 1970s, it gives some idea of the prevailing conditions in healthcare provision when, in the mid-1970s, we were generating our thoughts about the Roper-Logan-Tierney model of nursing. To focus a model of nursing on a model of *living* seemed particularly in keeping with the emergent trends in nursing and health care.

Development of the Roper-Logan-Tierney model of nursing

If a model can be said to have a place of origin, the Roper-Logan-Tierney model is indisputably from Edinburgh, Scotland. All three of the trio are graduates of the University of Edinburgh and all have worked and/or studied at that University's well-known Department of Nursing Studies at some time in their careers.

Before studying for a Master's degree at the University of Edinburgh, *Nancy Roper* left an established career as a nurse teacher to become self-employed as an author of nursing textbooks, and became internationally known as a lexicographer. Over a period of years, she had become concerned about the words used to describe nursing. For example, in the 1960s, student nurses were allocated to various wards to gain experience in medical, surgical, gynaecological, orthopaedic nursing and so on, as specialization in health care was ever increasing. There were also broader classifications such as paediatric nursing and psychiatric nursing.

So in 1970, as part of her Master's thesis, Roper started to investigate whether or not there was an identifiable 'core' of nursing across these various nursing specialties because, if such a core existed, it should be possible to identify not only the core, but also the specialized knowledge, skills and attitudes required to nurse people who had a gynaecological or an orthopaedic condition, and so on. Identification of a 'core', Roper postulated, would explicate the 'unity' of nursing, and identification of the particular knowledge and skills needed in the 'specialties' would explicate its 'diversity'.

There was a library search of other projects related to identification of a core of nursing, but none had been conducted in clinical areas. So a 'patient profile' was used to collect data from patients in all clinical areas to which one college of nursing allocated its students: one general hospital (which included long-stay beds), one maternity hospital, one psychiatric hospital and 12 community districts. The resulting 774 profiles were analysed and the results revealed that, clearly, there was a 'core' that related to everyday living activities, providing support for Roper's idea of basing a model of nursing on a model of living, and thereby acknowledging the indisputable fact that patients/clients have to continue 'living' while they are receiving nursing and, indeed, that nurses are engaged in living alongside their nursing. However, the original Roper models (Roper 1976) are now only of historical interest. The ideas from them were enlarged and regrouped to produce the Roper-Logan-Tierney model of nursing, based on a model of living.

Winifred Logan brought to the trio further experience as a nurse educator and, importantly, wide experience of nursing internationally. Logan had joined the staff of the Department of Nursing Studies at the University of Edinburgh in 1962; she already had a Master's degree from the University. It is not easy to pinpoint the experiences that contributed specifically to an interest in conceptual frameworks for nursing but, in retrospect, perhaps two are noteworthy.

While in Canada in the 1950s, Logan worked in a tuberculosis/thoracic unit where Inuits had been airlifted from Baffinland to Hamilton, Ontario. The 'culture shock' experienced on being rapidly transported from living in igloos or skin tents to life in a modern hospital can scarcely be imagined; the patients' reactions to illness and treatment within an alien environment provided staff with an extreme example of the importance of considering psychological, sociocultural and environmental factors, as well as the more obvious disease condition. Subsequently, when submitting the final dissertation for a teaching qualification at the University of Edinburgh in 1961, Logan chose to discuss 'Psychological and sociocultural aspects of nursing'. Later experience as a WHO consultant, as executive director of the International Council of Nurses, and when reflecting on the increasingly multicultural society in the UK, the importance of these aspects of nursing was underscored, irrespective of the client's health or disease status.

Another landmark was study for a Master's degree at Columbia University, New York, in the 1960s. Renowned pioneers who successfully articulated their thinking about the nature of nursing were products of Columbia University (e.g. Virginia Henderson, Hildegarde Peplau, Fay Abdellah and Lydia Hall), and in the 1960s models of nursing and all aspects of the nursing process were being hotly debated in the USA. Not surprisingly, when Logan returned to the staff of the University of Edinburgh, she used some of this content in her teaching, and in her thinking about the nature of nursing. So when Roper indicated that she wanted to develop her ideas about a model of nursing based on a model of living, which she published in 1976 as a monograph *Clinical Experience in Nurse Education*, Logan accepted the invitation to collaborate, along with Alison Tierney.

Alison Tierney was a young lecturer in the Department of Nursing Studies at the University of Edinburgh when invited to become the third member of the Roper-Logan-Tierney 'trio'. Roper had started her Master of Philosophy study in the Department when, in 1971, Tierney returned there to work for a Doctor of Philosophy degree, having previously undertaken the integrated nursing/degree programme during the time Logan was a course organizer of the programme and a senior lecturer in the department.

In the mid-1970s Tierney found the invitation to work with Roper and Logan on the development of a nursing model to be well timed: she was in the throes of restructuring the foundation course of the degree/nursing programme and immediately saw the potential value of organizing the course within the framework of a nursing model. Indeed, the Roper-Logan-Tierney model, even before its first publication, was being used very effectively as a means of drawing together previously disparate strands of teaching from the range of physical and social sciences into a coherent, nursing-centred, introductory course for students taking the degree/nursing programme.

Over time, Tierney's continuing contribution to the ongoing development of the model has drawn increasingly on her skills as a nurse researcher. Her role over a 10-year period (1984–1994) as director of the Nursing Research Unit (a national centre based at the University of Edinburgh) enabled Tierney to become involved in fostering the strategic development of nursing research at national and international levels through contacts with the National Centre (now Institute) for Nursing Research in the USA; work with the International Council of Nurses; and networking within the Workgroup of European Nurse Researchers on which she represented the UK on behalf of the Royal College of Nursing for much of the 1990s. Tierney now holds a Personal Chair in Nursing Research at the University of Edinburgh.

As research has flourished in nursing over the 1980s and 1990s, the inclusion of up-to-date research evidence to underpin the content of *The Elements of Nursing* has become an increasingly demanding task in each new edition of the book. It is almost impossible now to keep abreast with research relating to the range of subjects in the book, and particularly in relation to the 12 Activities of Living; as a result, parts of *The Elements of Nursing* are out of date almost as soon as a new edition is published. It is mainly for that reason that we decided not to produce another edition, but instead, to extract from the book *the model* that has been at the centre of our work from the outset, and in this more lasting form of publication (i.e. a monograph) to present an account of the model as it stands at the end of the 1990s. In the future, others may choose to refine the model further—as we ourselves have done over the years—or to adapt it, or even to incorporate it within a new and different model of nursing in response to the continuing changes that will reshape nursing and health care in the years to come.

REFERENCES

Aggleton P, Chalmers H 2000 Nursing models and the nursing process, 2nd edn. Macmillan, Basingstoke, UK

Fawcett J 1995 Conceptual models of nursing. F A Davis, Philadelphia

Henderson V 1960 The basic principles of nursing care. International Council of Nurses, Geneva

Marriner Tomey A, Alligood M 1998. Nursing theorists and their work, 4th edn. Mosby, St Louis

Meleis A 1997 Theoretical nursing: development and progress, 3rd edn. Lippincott, Philadelphia

Roper N 1976 Clinical experience in nurse education. Churchill Livingstone, Edinburgh

Roper N, Logan W, Tierney A 1980, 1985, 1990, 1996 The elements of nursing, 1st, 2nd, 3rd, 4th edn. Churchill Livingstone, Edinburgh

The model of living

To encapsulate the complexities of 'living' in a model that is simple enough to be meaningful is, of course, impossible. 'Living', although having obvious physical manifestations, some of which lend themselves to objective description, also has many other dimensions. The current understanding of living is not at all complete, but knowledge available from the natural sciences, the social sciences and the humanities does give an insight into the nature of living. So it is inevitable that, despite commonalities, each reader's concept of living may differ in a number of aspects and, indeed, may change over time.

The model of living that underpins the Roper-Logan-Tierney model of nursing is an attempt to identify only the main features of this highly complex phenomenon. As indicated in Figure 2.1 we include five main components (concepts) in our model and, very importantly, the concepts are interrelated:

- Activities of Living (ALs)
- Lifespan
- Dependence/independence continuum
- Factors influencing ALs

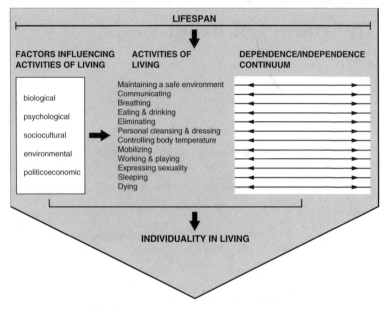

Figure 2.1 The model of living.

● Individuality in living.

In the following text, each of the concepts of the model of living will be discussed in turn. The definition of the term 'concept' and Fawcett's definition of a conceptual model are given in Boxes 2.1 and 2.2, respectively, and we have adopted these in the construction of our models.

Box 2.1 Definition of a concept

CONCEPT
A concept is a word symbol, a symbolic representation for a class of objects.
A concept:

● permits generalization
● is a means of organizing and classifying data
● is an economical way of storing and using a mass of discrete pieces of data.

A concept cannot be taught as such; it is developed by each person as a system of learned responses provided by sense perceptions.

Box 2.2 Definition of a conceptual model

CONCEPTUAL MODEL
Fawcett (1995) uses the following definition:

a set of abstract and general concepts and the propositions (statements which link concepts) that integrate these concepts into a meaningful configuration.

Activities of Living (ALs)

A model of living must offer a way of describing what 'living' means. If asked to describe what everyday living involves, most people—irrespective of their age and circumstances—would mention activities such as eating and drinking, working and playing, and sleeping. If prompted, they would probably agree that breathing and communicating are also activities that are an integral part of living, even if at times they seem to be performed without much conscious deliberation. All of these activities, and others, such as eliminating, maintaining a safe environment, and personal cleansing and dressing, collectively contribute to the complex process of living. They are *activities of living*.

It is this concept that is used as the focus of our model of living, and after much deliberation and discussion between ourselves and with others, we translated it for practical purposes into a set of ALs, 12 in number (Fig. 2.2). It is the central component of the

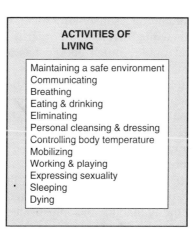

ACTIVITIES OF LIVING

Maintaining a safe environment
Communicating
Breathing
Eating & drinking
Eliminating
Personal cleansing & dressing
Controlling body temperature
Mobilizing
Working & playing
Expressing sexuality
Sleeping
Dying

Figure 2.2 The Activities of Living.

model. The lifespan, the dependence/independence continuum, and the influencing factors are all interpreted in terms of their relationship to each of the 12 ALs. These four interacting concepts (ALs, lifespan, dependence/independence continuum, factors) combine to produce the unique mix that determines the fifth concept: individuality in living.

The term 'Activity of Living' is used as an all-embracing one. Each 'Activity' has many dimensions; indeed, it could be thought of as an overall activity composed of a number of particular activities, rather as a compound is made up of a number of elements. The more one analyses the ALs, the more one realizes just how complex each one is. Compounding this complexity is the fact that they are so closely related. For example, communicating is related to many of the other ALs: just imagine eating and drinking, working and playing, and expressing sexuality without communicating! And breathing is essential for all of the ALs. So, only for the purpose of description and learning can they be separated, and here only a very brief description of each AL is necessary by way of introduction and to give the general flavour of what are enormously complex concepts. In no way are these presented as comprehensive descriptions of the 12 ALs; they are short sketches which serve merely to emphasize the complexity of each AL.

The AL of maintaining a safe environment

Every day people are engaged in many activities with the specific purpose of maintaining a safe environment, whether at home, at work, at play or while travelling. In order to maintain health, both personal and public, much energy has to be directed at maintaining an environment that is as safe as possible, not only for the present but for future generations to inherit.

Throughout history, humankind has been concerned with controlling the external environment or adapting to its vagaries. To an amazing degree humans have conquered the dangers inherent in the physical environment and have devised methods of protecting their family, property, crops and livestock. Nowadays, most humans no longer live in constant threat of danger, although there are powerful natural forces that they are impotent to control despite the availability of sophisticated technology. The fact that this is the case is illustrated by events in recent history, such as earthquakes, devastating forest fires, the virtually annual floods in the Indian subcontinent in the wake of the monsoon rains, and the continuing drought in parts of the African continent which have taken the lives and livelihood of countless people. It should not be forgotten either that, in this so-called era of peace, there are wars going on in many parts of the world which means that some people are living in an unsafe environment and in constant danger. Increasingly too, with ongoing technological and scientific advancement, there are yet new hazards to contend with—such as risks associated with radiation, chemical waste, the illicit use of drugs and modern war weaponry—and these, in contrast to natural forces, have been created by humans themselves.

Potential hazards. Even under normal circumstances, however, people throughout the world are still exposed to a variety of environmental hazards that jeopardize their safety, health and, indeed, survival.

External agents. A variety of external agents in the environment —at home, at school, in the workplace and in recreational settings —can cause injury, disease or infection. The body of a healthy person has a remarkable ability to counter such assaults via mechanisms such as the skeletal protection of vital organs; cilia in the respiratory tract to hasten the exit of harmful foreign material from the lungs; the secretion of tears to protect the eye; the powerful immune system; the body's ability to regenerate damaged tissue. However, the injury, disease or infection may overwhelm these body defences, and more serious illness or death may ensue.

Stress. Excessive stress is increasingly recognized as a form of environmental hazard. As well as biological stressors, there are more subtle psychological and sociocultural stressors, sometimes associated with life events such as weaning, puberty, or even the varying degree of pleasurability–sadness surrounding incidents such as changing school, job or house; getting married or divorced; childbearing; and the death of loved ones. Psychological stressors are known to be important in relation to the incidence of accidents in all age groups, and excessive stress may have mental and physical repercussions in varying degrees.

Abuse. The environment is anything but safe when there is physical or emotional or sexual abuse of children; of women; of elderly people; or of disabled people. Nowadays, there is much more public awareness of the lasting physical and mental harm suffered by such vulnerable victims of abuse.

Social disorder. An alarming threat to safety in the environment, which is a disturbing feature of modern living, is the increase in social disorder, which occurs across social boundaries. There is a rising tide of purposeless thuggery and vandalism, and not only adults are involved; at school, quite young children indulge in bullying (peer abuse), physical violence to fellow pupils and teachers, and sometimes even murder. Quite apart from identifying the perpetrators of such crimes, there is much more public demand to support the victims, who may suffer persistent adverse symptoms, now recognized as post-traumatic stress disorder (PTSD). Even related to religion and spirituality there can be a form of violence or disorder resulting in the death of adherents or, in other instances, the death of innocent people. When adherents leave these new style cults or are 'rescued', exit counselling or even deprogramming is often required, and the mental health of the ex-adherent may be in jeopardy.

Preventing potential hazards. Dissemination of knowledge about many aspects of safety in the environment and the prevention of hazards is undertaken via health education programmes at school and at work as well as by publicity programmes and television documentaries. The general gist of these efforts is to attempt to change attitudes and behaviour in a positive way. And in many countries, of course, there are legal requirements to promote safety, for example: to regulate traffic (land, sea and air) and thus prevent accidents; to prevent contamination by waste materials, chemicals and nuclear products; to ensure that protective clothing is worn in the workplace when there are known hazards; to apprehend people who engage in bullying, harassment and violence; to ensure that there are high standards of hygiene in the commercial handling of foodstuffs in order to prevent infection; to be protective and supportive to vulnerable people who are experiencing severe mental disturbance and need professional care as outlined in Mental Health Acts.

Obviously a vast array of professionals, employers and officials is involved in maintaining a safe environment for the general public, and each individual also has to accept a personal responsibility for their own safety.

Of course, these are only a few examples of the scores of activities that could be included in a discussion about the AL of maintaining a safe environment.

The AL of communicating

Humans are essentially social beings and spend the major part of each day communicating with other people. The activity of communicating is therefore an integral part of all human relationships and all human behaviour. Indeed, any information given or received about all the other ALs is via communicating in one form or another.

The process of communicating. The study of cybernetics has contributed considerably to the understanding of the process of communicating. As long ago as 1960, in a classic work, Berlo proposed a model of communication, consisting of four components: source, message, channel and receiver. Communication is said to occur when a person (the source) sends a message in a particular medium (channel) so that it is received by a recipient (receiver). This process has been adapted to form a two-way model in which the communication elicits a response in the receiver. The response, in turn, causes the receiver to become the source of a return message, which is sent via a chosen channel, thus providing feedback to the original source (Fig. 2.3).

Broadly speaking, communicating generally utilizes two main channels: 'verbal' and 'non-verbal'. Verbal communication consists of the spoken or written word, whereas non-verbal communication includes paralanguage and kinetics, but of course often they are used simultaneously (Fig. 2.3). Wiggens et al (1994) use the term 'paralanguage' to define the non-semantic aspects of verbal communication which we use to express the meaning that our words convey. Paralanguage concerns how we use language, rather than what we say. It includes the tone of voice, the speed with which we speak and our use of 'filler' sounds such as 'um' and 'er'. Such communication can be said to be vocal rather than verbal.

The study of non-verbal communication or body language is now receiving much more attention, and the term 'kine' has been adopted for each 'unit' of body movement that transmits a message. The kine is analogous to a letter in the verbal alphabet. Kinetics is still a young science, but it would seem that the human ability to exert conscious control over body language is less than with verbal communication, and most people, at times, are aware of sending contradictory messages.

Non-verbal communication serves a number of purposes depending on the context. The whole body may be conveying a

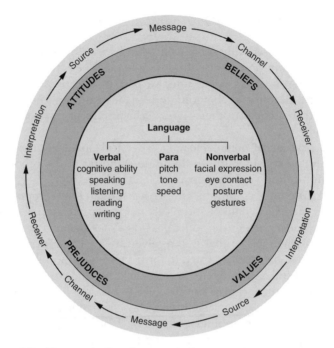

Figure 2.3 The complexities of communicating.

message. Humans use their bodies to express themselves, for instance in the way they walk. Walking boldly into a room may be indicative of a feeling of well-being; on the other hand it may be conveying a mood of anger. Walking slowly into a room may indicate reticence or apprehension. The stance that people take, too, can transmit an impression as varied as boredom, exhaustion, attentiveness and interest.

Facial expression is a rich source of information regarding the emotional state of the individual. One can transmit impressions such as disapproval, disgust, anger, irritation, pleasure, love and understanding by facial gesture; indeed, its effectiveness is recognized in colloquial expressions such as 'a look enough to kill' or 'a sour look'. The eyes can be particularly revealing, and people vary in the amount of eye contact they make and maintain while communicating, and this can be culturally determined.

Hands are especially important to body language, usually to provide points of emphasis, while shaping with the hands the object being discussed, or an event, or signalling directions.

Hands also convey emotion, for example reflecting inner anxiety by restless, wringing movements or fiddling with small objects; or anger when showing white knuckles or clenched fists.

It is apparent that physical appearance and presence are powerful aspects of non-verbal communication, and the variety of make-up products, jewellery, perfume, aftershave and spectacle frames in department stores is an eloquent reflection of the range of taste. Clothes, too, although essentially intended to protect from the elements, provide a great deal of information about the wearer. They can express current mood, state of finance, preparation to take part in sport, or to go to work. Indeed the term 'language of clothes' is quite commonly used and is related to the AL of personal cleansing and dressing, and to the AL of expressing sexuality.

Communicating by touch can be a powerful way of relaying a message; indeed it is usually associated with more intimate relationships. Therapeutic or 'conscious' touch may be used deliberately, however, often conveying sympathy while communicating verbally with someone who has a problem, or when conveying bad news. But there are considerable cultural differences related to 'touching' and the user must be discerning when employing this mode of communicating.

Circumstances that influence communicating. Obviously *age* is a crucial factor in relation to communicating. Decoding the communicating activities of babies and children, both verbally and non-verbally, requires patience and skill. The young are certainly dependent on others for help with this AL, and likewise some elderly people. For quite different reasons, people with certain mental health problems, with specific physical disabilities, and with major learning difficulties may also be dependent on others for help.

It goes without saying, that biological *body structure* related to sight, hearing, smell and taste is basic to independence in communicating although some degree of impairment may be compensated for by using, for example, a hearing aid or spectacles—a form of 'aided' independence.

Inevitably, *level of intelligence* affects communicating in that it influences learning ability and memory for vocabulary used in speech, and also for the acts of listening, writing and reading. Yet no matter how fluent in the use of vocabulary, a person's emotion and *current mood* also have an effect on this AL (e.g.

excitement, depression, level of self-esteem and concept of body image).

Quite often, the person's *social and cultural values* will influence this AL (Fig. 2.3); indeed, there may be miscommunication related to racial or ethnic differences quite apart from language problems, especially when technical or specialist vocabulary is being used. Such problems are exacerbated when the environment for communicating is unhelpful—too noisy, too warm or cold, inadequate lighting.

Technological advances. Of course, technological advances have greatly enhanced the capacity to communicate via the mass media, telephone, fax, e-mail, the Internet and facilities for using, for example, teleconferencing and telemedicine. However, with such advances come ethical concerns about confidentiality and ease of data retrieval in organizations associated with, for example, commerce, government, education and health services. Data Protection Acts attempt to ensure confidentiality but determined abusers of such systems seem to be able, on occasion, to circumvent legal requirements.

Communicating is a highly individual activity. Yet, in discussing communicating, it is not the individual who is crucial, but the interpersonal relationship. To understand this AL, one has to understand how people relate to one another. There are many aspects to this vast subject of communicating, and the above comments merely provide a general outline which, if anything, serves to emphasize its complexities.

The AL of breathing

'Taking the first breath' is of crucial importance at the birth of every baby and determines whether or not the infant will have a viable existence as a human being. From then on, breathing seems effortless and people are not usually consciously aware of the AL of breathing until some abnormal circumstance forces it to their attention.

Respiratory–cardiovascular link. The organs that collectively form the respiratory system provide every cell in the body with oxygen via the processes known as external and internal respiration. To accomplish this, the blood, together with the vessels and organs comprising the circulatory and lymphatic systems, is also required. So, breathing involves the respiratory system and also the cardiovascular system.

During vigorous exercise in the healthy adult there is a normal physiological increase in respiratory rate, because the muscles require more oxygen. To transport the oxygen more quickly, the heart beats faster so the pulse rate is simultaneously increased; in fact, respiration and pulse rates are related in a ratio of 1:4, and an alteration in one is usually accompanied by an alteration in the other. Conversely, when the body is resting, particularly when sleeping, the respiratory rate and pulse rate are usually decreased.

Not only rate but also rhythm of breathing can be affected during physical activities such as talking, laughing, eating and singing, yet seldom are these variations given conscious thought. Even sneezing and coughing, if transient, are rarely pondered over as a deviation in the normal pattern of breathing.

Emotional aspects. Emotional events in life can also affect the individual's breathing. Sadness and grieving may influence the rate and depth of respirations, resulting in audible and visible activities such as sighing and sobbing. And, in response to perceived danger, the body reacts by increasing the rate and depth of respiration, as well as the heart rate, blood pressure and flow of blood to the muscles. In extreme form, these increases are part of the 'fight or flight' syndromes that facilitate survival. However, for most of the time, reaction to fear is much less intense.

Anxiety causes the body to react in a similar way, physiologically, and, although less intense in the short term, is frequently of much longer duration. Everyone experiences anxiety in one form or another at some time in their lives, but a period of prolonged anxiety is undesirable. Some people can be helped to overcome its effects by engaging in simple relaxation techniques, many of which involve controlled breathing as practised, for example, in chanting, transcendental meditation and yoga. Currently there is interest in helping tense people to relax and lower their blood pressure and pulse rates by visual technological monitoring of these functions. However, the part played by temperament and emotion is difficult to assess and there is no doubt that worry about high blood pressure readings is likely to exacerbate the problem.

Potential hazards

Tobacco smoke. It is now widely accepted that breathing is influenced by smoking, which adversely affects the tissue in the respiratory system but is also detrimental to the integrity of the cardiovascular system. The carbon monoxide (CO) in tobacco smoke binds with haemoglobin in red blood cells to form carboxyhaemoglobin, which does not easily exchange oxygen. Consequently there is a reduction in the oxygen-carrying capacity of the blood, so it is understandable that there may be widespread effects throughout the body. In many countries, considerable effort is made to educate people to refrain from adopting the habit, or to give up what becomes, insidiously, a form of social dependence. The adverse effects of 'passive smoking' when living or working in a smoke-filled atmosphere are controversial. It certainly is considered to be unpleasant by most non-smokers, and in many public places, on transport and in work settings, smoking is now prohibited.

Pathogens. Atmospheric air is a mixture of gases and has variable humidity but it also contains microorganisms. In the air, there are many millions of microorganisms; most are non-pathogenic but some, when inhaled, cause infection of the respiratory tract, for example the common cold. In varying degrees, such infections affect the rate, depth and rhythm of breathing. Indoors, these pathogens fall to the floor or settle on household objects by force of gravity, and convection currents promote their circulation in the atmosphere, so perpetuating the possibility of inhalation and further infection.

Pollutants. At home, householders may pollute the air by failing to provide good ventilation, thus increasing the concentration of products from expired air. The carbon dioxide content does not necessarily reach dangerous levels but the increased temperature and humidity is conducive to rapid multiplication of pathogens. Also, if poorly ventilated, the inhalation of any gases leaking from appliances and from paraffin stoves can cause headaches, drowsiness or indeed, in large quantity, may render the occupants unconscious.

In the work environment, there may be exposure to respiratory abrasion from industrial waste particles, organic and inorganic, for example from linen, hemp, wool, metal, stone and coal. The coal-mining industry, for example, has a long history of protective practices to prevent the onset of the dreaded disease, pneumoconiosis, which develops when coal-dust particles become embedded in the lung tissue and eventually cause gross impairment in the capacity to breathe. Workers who are at risk in these types of industries are encouraged to use the appropriate preventive measures provided and to have regular chest X-rays so that any adverse effects will be promptly detected and treated. At an international level, the International Labour Organization (ILO) has taken measures to encourage governments to provide employees with protection from several types of respiratory health hazards.

While out of doors, especially in and around an urban area, people are frequently exposed to possible abrasion of the tissue in the respiratory tract by inhalation of smoke containing minute particles which are the products of combustion in domestic heating systems, industrial establishments and transport vehicles. The problem of atmospheric pollution is primarily a responsibility of government, and in many industrialized countries legislation exists to control and reduce the associated hazards, especially for city dwellers and workers at risk. The generation of power by means of fossil fuels is a major atmospheric pollutant in many parts of the world and the potential for alternatives such as solar, wind or wavepower is being explored with varying degrees of success. However, individuals have responsibilities too, for example to comply with the requirement to burn smokeless fuel or to wear a protective breathing mask when engaged in certain types of work. By so doing, individuals minimize the risks to others and avoid hazards that might affect their own breathing.

At an international level, the World Health Organization (WHO) is studying and monitoring the problem of atmospheric pollution and assisting with the exchange of information about prevention on a worldwide scale so that the air, so important to the AL of breathing and so necessary to human life, will be less of a health hazard. All the ALs are entirely dependent on the AL of breathing.

The AL of eating and drinking

Eating and drinking play a significant part in the everyday living pattern of all age groups, and for most people they are pleasurable activities. But, apart from the pleasure derived, eating and drinking are essential to existence. The human body is a highly complex collection of millions of cells, and the cycle of each cell's growth and development, as well as the constant cell activity, requires an energy source: it is obtained from the body's food and fluid intake.

At subsistence level, human beings will eat almost any food, often in its raw state, in order to meet the basic need for sustenance. Normally, however, provided that an adequate, well-balanced diet is available, food and fluid intake is regulated by complex biochemical processes. In the brain there are centres that control appetite and thirst; they are sensitive to changes in the level of nutrients and fluid in the blood. A visible physical dimension resulting from eating and drinking is body size; height and weight are measurable physical data.

The study of food, and the associated biological processes of the growth, maintenance and repair of body tissue, is the science of nutrition, and the unit for dietetic calculation is the calorie, or, if using the Système International, the kilojoule. The kilojoule requirement for an individual varies with height, weight, age, sex, climate and occupation.

Intellectual and emotional variations. There are many dimensions to the AL of eating and drinking apart from the physical intake of food and fluid. A minimal level of intelligence is needed to acquire the skills used in the act of eating and drinking. This is apparent when observing young children as they experiment intellectually as well as physically with mealtime skills, and, similarly, it is apparent when observing people whose intellectual development has been impaired: they often have great difficulty in acquiring such skills. A certain intellectual development is also required for the acquisition and application of the knowledge needed to select and prepare a diet that will maintain health. Currently, a great deal of effort is expended by health professionals, government agencies and the media on health education in order to interest the general public about desirable eating practices. The acquisition of knowledge is required also to apply appropriate hygienic practices when handling food, and to dispose of food waste in such a manner that it will not attract vermin and flies, which have the potential to spread pathogens to humans. In many countries, there are strict legal requirements about the hygienic preparation of food that is sold commercially, and about the labelling of food additives. Indeed, when food manufacturers appear to be meddling with food safety, a better-educated and now better-informed buyer is more willing to express public outrage, as shown, for example, when genetically modified foods were marketed without—it seemed—adequate consultation about long-term effects on health.

The individual's emotional state, too, may affect food intake. The child's excitement before a holiday, the anxiety associated with examinations, the stress of a change of job may well reduce the accustomed intake for the individual. But these are usually transient variations. Loss of appetite or lack of desire for food over a prolonged period can be indicators of a more serious disturbance of the emotional state, as is seen in anorexia nervosa which has its peak incidence in adolescence, especially among young women.

However, in contradistinction, some people may use food as a source of comfort and security, and this overeating may lead to obesity. Some overweight people are quite comfortable with their body image but others may choose to diet and some may be advised to lose excessive weight, for example if arthritis develops in the lower limbs. Bulimia nervosa with its 'binge eating' is another example of an overeating disturbance. Overdrinking may also be a problem. The frequent overconsumption of alcoholic beverages—sometimes a negative coping mechanism in response to emotional disturbance—is a major concern in many countries of the world, often leading to irresponsible behaviour or even crime, and causing much distress not only to the individual, but also to family and friends.

Sociocultural variations. Quite apart from the nutrient content of food, a meal provides an opportunity for the young child to learn about the rituals related to serving food, and they begin to appreciate that food can have considerable social significance concerned with interpersonal relationships. In almost all cultures, offering a meal to visitors is one overt way of expressing friendship and hospitality, and in almost all societies eating and drinking are an integral part of such diverse family occasions as birth, marriage and death, and also of some national holidays and religious festivals.

Religion, too, may have a considerable influence on eating and drinking practices. Certain religious groups have definite rules about the choice and preparation of specific items on the menu; for example, orthodox Jews must prepare and serve dairy products and meat dishes separately, while the Koran forbids Muslims to touch pork or alcohol, and the devout Hindu will not eat animal products.

Availability of food and drink. It is not difficult to appreciate that the physical environment can affect the choice of food. Obviously geographical position, soil fertility, climate and rainfall will determine the type of food that can be grown locally, and will also influence the meat, fish and poultry content of the diet; nowadays, for industrialized nations with their extensive import–export networks, reliance on local food is not such a dominant feature of everyday living, but it is crucial for about two-thirds of the world who are dependent on local produce.

For most people, any considerations of eating and drinking presupposes that food and drink are available, but in certain areas of the world many thousands are dying because of under-nourishment or lack of a safe water supply. There are many complex reasons for this maldistribution. Considerable attempts have been made at national and international levels to redress these gross inequalities but still the problem remains, much of it due to economic and political constraints.

With the interaction of so many variables, it is not surprising that each person develops deep-rooted beliefs and attitudes about food, as well as individual patterns related to the AL of eating and drinking.

The AL of eliminating

Eliminating is an activity of living that all individuals perform with unfailing regularity throughout life. Whatever people are doing, wherever they are, and regardless of the time of day, they respond to the need to eliminate, and this response is an integral activity of everyday life. Throughout the world, people are socialized into eliminating in private and this contributes to many strongly held attitudes and taboos associated with this AL. In public buildings, and even in the family home, the provision of a place affording privacy to the individual for eliminating is usually considered to be essential. Even in societies that emphasize the communal nature of ALs, eliminating is normally a private activity and the products of elimination are concealed from the public eye.

So essential is eliminating that even unicellular organisms must rid themselves of waste products from metabolic processes. In many multicellular organisms, however, separate systems deal with the elimination of waste products. We have chosen to describe urinary and faecal elimination together because, although two distinct body systems are involved, there is no good reason to separate them in the context of an AL framework.

The main purpose of eliminating *urine* is to dispose of unrequired fluid intake and dissolved chemicals which the body cells are not immediately requiring (and which cannot be stored) so that the body is correctly hydrated, in an electrolyte balance and thereby in overall acid–base balance. Urine is secreted throughout the 24 hours, but production slows during sleep, and voiding is usually unnecessary during that period; so the first urine voided on waking is normally darker in colour owing to its concentration. Otherwise the colour ranges from amber to straw-coloured. Urine has a relative density of between 1.015 and 1.025, and is normally acidic with a pH of about 6. It is composed of about 96% water, 2% salts (especially sodium and potassium) and 2% nitrogenous waste (urea). When recently voided, it has only a slight smell, but after exposure to air it decomposes and begins to smell of ammonia. A high fluid intake results in a high urine output, and vice versa. However, the normal urine output is around 1 to 1.1/2 litres in 24 hours; the usual frequency of micturition is between 5 and 10 times in that period.

The main purpose of excreting *faeces* is to rid the body of indigestible cellulose and unabsorbed food, but faeces also contain shed endothelial cells, intestinal secretions, water and bacteria. The first stool of the infant is a sticky greenish-black substance (meconium) containing amniotic fluid, bile pigments and fats. Meconium is passed several times in the first few days of life. Then a brownish-green stool is passed and, a few days later, the baby's excreta become yellow in colour. A breast-fed baby has softer, brighter yellow stools than a bottle-fed baby, whose stools are pale, more formed and with a slightly offensive smell. Once the infant is weaned and beginning to have a balanced diet of normal foodstuffs, the faeces begin to take on their familiar composition. Faecal matter in the adult is normally brown in colour, soft in consistency and cylindrical in form. There is an odour from faeces due to the action of bacterial flora in the intestine; the smell varies according to the bacteria present and the type of food ingested. Faeces are normally composed of water (75%) and solid matter (25%) made up of quantities of dead bacteria, some fatty acids, inorganic matter, proteins and undigested dietary fibre.

With regard to number and size of stools, people in Western societies, on average, excrete one stool daily, weighing around 80–120 g.

Activities associated with eliminating. To be able to eliminate in the normal way requires fully functioning urinary and defaecatory systems along with their related sensory and motor nerve supply. The infant and young child eliminates waste products by a reflex involuntary action and, depending on cultural customs, is kept in a clean and dry state by the mother or older people. As the nerve supply matures, a voluntary control becomes possible, and the young child is socialized into the activities associated with eliminating, usually in privacy. At the other end of the lifespan, the urinary and defaecatory systems sometimes become less efficient with reduced muscle tone, and the older person may experience incontinence, bringing with it all the embarrassment and loss of dignity which that entails.

Obviously, the AL of eliminating involves more than the physical acts of micturition and defaecation. The person must be able to reach the toilet, adjust clothing, sit and rise from the toilet, use toilet tissue, and wash their hands. In some religions and cultural groups, post-elimination hygiene is strictly prescribed but, of course, it is desirable that everyone is socialized into using safe hygiene practices related to eliminating in order to prevent the spread of infection, particularly diarrhoeal infections. Clearly the AL of eliminating is closely related to the AL of mobilizing and to the AL of personal cleansing and dressing.

Sometimes, however, physical and intellectual control are superseded by *emotional influences*; for example, most people have experienced the urgent need to empty their bladder when facing a stressful situation such as an examination. On the other hand, depression is often associated with apathy and sluggishness, and this may influence eliminating, resulting in constipation.

Facilities associated with eliminating. It is all too easy for those accustomed to flushing toilets (attached to a water carriage system of sewage disposal) to think that these are the norm. But in some parts of the world people are fortunate to have a chemical toilet, or indeed an earth toilet, because in some other places there are no amenities—people 'go into the bush' to defaecate. These waste products prove an immediate attraction for flies and, especially if close to a cluster of human habitations, are one of the vehicles for transmitting infection to food and causing diarrhoeal diseases. Many developing countries have an inordinately high mortality rate from diarrhoeal disease, especially among children. Although economic aid from a variety of international sources is sometimes used to encourage villagers to construct simple earth toilets—in an attempt to control the exposure of human waste products and thus reduce morbidity and mortality rates—there are varying degrees of success.

From time to time, following major natural disasters such as earthquakes and extensive flooding, the need for emergency sanitation is essential. Relief workers attempt to provide emergency facilities to deal safely with the products of elimination in order to prevent the spread of diarrhoeal infection among large numbers of people who are already homeless and in acute distress.

In the West, people take so much for granted. They scarcely give a thought to the many advantages that modern sanitation systems provide in relation to the very necessary and daily AL of eliminating.

The AL of personal cleansing and dressing

Throughout the ages people have paid attention to personal hygiene; indeed, there is archaeological evidence of the means whereby these activities were performed by members of previous civilizations. In each historical period there has been a gradual refinement of the articles used for cleansing the skin, hair, nails and teeth. Today, the ever-increasing advertising of the cosmetic and hairdressing industries has increased most people's interest in personal grooming.

The clothing and fashion industries have developed equally expansively. Clothes today are very different from those in past times; clothing worn by members of previous generations on formal occasions is evident from paintings, and also depicted are the clothes worn for leisure-time activities and for different types of work. Currently progress in manufacturing processes has resulted in a wide variety of 'easy-care' clothes for every conceivable occasion, so that people can now enjoy this part of everyday living with less effort and greater variety.

The objective in most cultures is to socialize children into independent performance of personal cleansing and dressing activities, usually in privacy and in rooms set aside for these purposes. For most people the attitude is inculcated from an early age that cleansing and clothing one's body is a personal concern, which if not carried out in privacy is usually accomplished only in the presence of close family members. But the end result is observable by others, cleanliness and good grooming being commended in most cultures, while lack of these is deplored, particularly if accompanied by malodour and infestation.

Daily hygiene. There are several activities associated with personal cleansing. Most people clean the *skin* by washing with soap and water, rinsing and drying. It may be an 'all-over' wash using a basin of water, an immersion bath or a shower. However it is accomplished, children are socialized by membership of the family into a frequency norm for this 'all-over' cleansing, such as daily or weekly.

Everyone is now encouraged to wash their hands before preparing or eating food and after visiting the toilet. *Handwashing* is undoubtedly the main activity in preventing the spread of infection in the home, at work and in recreational settings, as well as at clinics and in hospitals. The bacterial flora of the hands is similar to that of other skin sites, but hands are of specific significance in the transmission of infectious agents and are the most important site of contamination. Most *resident skin flora* are not highly virulent and are not normally implicated in infections. In contrast, *transient flora* from an already infected site are frequently involved in cross-infection. *Finger and toe nails* are often cleaned and trimmed or manicured as part of the daily hygiene regimen and, for some people, the use of nail varnish may be an important aspect of adornment, and of expressing sexuality.

The moist membranes of the *female perineal area* require special attention to maintain health and comfort and to avoid malodour; this is especially important during the menstrual period. Females are encouraged to cleanse this area from front to back after elimination, especially of faeces. Microbiological data have confirmed that the majority of the infections of the female bladder (cystitis) are caused by microorganisms that normally inhabit the bowel and are present in faeces, and may therefore be in close proximity to the short urethra. Although these organisms are harmless in their natural habitat, they can be pathogenic in other organs of the body.

Many of the cells of the human body, if damaged, can be replaced but not the teeth—at least not the second growth of teeth. Following ingestion of food, especially sugars and refined carbohydrates, plaque builds up, adheres to the surface of teeth, is not easily removed and can lead to dental caries. So a rigorous routine of *teeth and mouth care* is essential. Ideally, food debris should be removed from teeth after each meal but a 3-minute brushing, at least once a day, is certainly recommended. It is known that fluoride protects teeth and is present in some water supplies or may be added to others; it is also an ingredient of many commercially produced toothpastes. But, in spite of improved knowledge about the causes and prevention, there is an increased incidence of dental caries in many countries and a lowering of the average age at which people become edentulous and require dentures. For some people, halitosis is a disturbing problem, and the individual may or may not be aware of their malodorous breath. A full dental and oral assessment is necessary and specialist treatment may be required.

Most people indulge in daily combing and/or brushing of the *hair*. Of all the personal cleansing activities, hair grooming has now become the least 'private', often undertaken in a hairdressing salon. To cater for every type of hair, there are numerous lotions, colourings and shampoos; hair styles, which change with the fashion, are an important aspect of self-image, and of expressing sexuality.

Variations in the skin, hair, nails and teeth that occur in the normal process of ageing give rise to differences in physical appearance at various stages in the lifespan. In turn, people modify, for example, make-up to suit skin changes, and alter hair styles as hair changes in condition and thickness.

Dressing. Changes in tradition and culture are reflected in clothes, and each succeeding generation modifies dress to suit the current environment and social conditions. In today's fast-moving world, it is expected that clothes will be easy to launder, and require minimal pressing and ironing.

Clothes are a medium of non-verbal communication. They can signify ethnic origin, level of income and social status, as well as personal preference for colour, style and fashion. They can also convey mood: when well, people usually maintain their clothes in good condition; when dejected, they do not seem to notice staining and lack of grooming.

Appropriate selection of clothes can reduce strain on the body's heat-regulating centre by protecting against rain, wind, cold, heat and sun, and can also protect from injury (e.g. the use of crash helmets). However, most people dress for personal adornment and derive great satisfaction from doing so. The activity of dressing offers the opportunity for making decisions that help to develop a feeling of self-direction, an important part of self- fulfilment, and a fascinating feature of the AL of expressing sexuality. So, clothes are a powerful vehicle of communication.

Reduced independence in choice. Obviously an individual's level of physical ability will determine the extent to which the various activities involved in personal cleansing and dressing can be carried out adequately; people who are physically disabled may have difficulty with some aspects of this AL. Some are so severely disabled that they cannot participate in any aspect of this AL and may be greatly frustrated by this constraint on their independence in such a private and personal activity of living. For quite different reasons, people who have a learning disability, and are by definition slow to learn, may require patient and repeated teaching in order to gain confidence and optimal independence in personal cleansing and dressing activities.

Personal income, of course, determines the amount of money that can be spent on basic items such as soap and other toiletries, and also restricts the amount of clothing that can be purchased. For those who are impoverished, clothing becomes simply a matter of necessity and the person is denied the pleasure of wearing attractive clothes and enjoying variety in dressing.

The AL of controlling body temperature

Unlike the cold-blooded animals whose temperature fluctuates according to the changing temperature of their external environment, humans are able to maintain body temperature at a constant level, independent of the degree of heat or cold in the surrounding environment. For most of the time people are unaware of their body temperature because it remains constantly at a comfortable level. This control of temperature is accomplished because a regulating centre in the hypothalamus of the brain carefully balances the amount of heat produced and lost by the body.

This balance is crucial. Most of the numerous biochemical processes occurring within the human body can take place only if the temperature of the body remains at a fairly constant level and within a relatively narrow range. The functioning of the nervous system is easily disturbed by temperatures outwith that narrow range of normal, and many other systems of the body are also adversely affected. Eventually, if the body temperature rises or falls excessively, there is permanent damage to body cells and the possibility of death. So essential is thermoregulation to health and survival that the body's own physiological control mechanisms are finely tuned.

Thermoregulation. In terms of physiological control of body temperature, the key factors are the temperature-regulating centre, heat production and heat loss.

Temperature regulation. An area of nerve tissue in the anterior part of the hypothalamus of the brain acts as a centre that regulates body temperature. Nerve cells in this area respond to changes in the temperature of circulating blood. It is thought that the centre also responds to impulses from the temperature-senstive receptors in the skin, muscles, blood vessels, the abdominal cavity and various areas of the central nervous system. The centre's function is to balance the amount of heat lost by the body. It works like a thermostat: there is a constant 'set' temperature which is maintained as the centre responds by balancing heat production and heat loss. To achieve this, the centre has two control mechanisms: its *heat-promoting centre* activates processes that increase heat production and reduce heat loss; conversely its *heat-losing centre* stimulates actions that reduce heat production and increase heat loss. These two centres work reciprocally; when one is activated, the other is depressed (Fig. 2.4).

Heat production. All the metabolic processes continuously occurring in the human body produce heat. At rest and during sleep the body is kept warm enough by the amount of energy produced at the basal metabolic rate. Additional heat production results mainly from skeletal muscle movement and, if this is not sufficient, the body initiates reflex muscular activity—shivering—which increases the rate of heat production up to fourfold. At the same time, stimulation of the sympathetic nervous system speeds up the process of cellular metabolism and raises the hairs on the skin, a vestigial mechanism in humans, which in hairier mammals traps the warm air next to the body, thereby insulating it. The prevention of unnecessary heat loss is an important way of conserving body heat. Most heat loss occurs through the skin by evaporation, conduction, convection and radiation. Vasoconstriction minimizes this heat loss because less warm

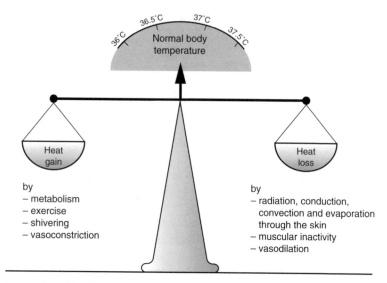

Figure 2.4 Heat loss–gain balance.

blood circulates in the subcutaneous tissue. At the same time, sweating is greatly diminished, reducing the amount of heat lost by evaporation.

Heat loss. A variety of means is used by the human body to lose heat. Heat is lost from skin that is in direct contact with cooler air by the process of conduction; this is assisted by convection currents of air circulating around the body. Heat is also lost by evaporation of moisture from the skin surface, naturally increased by sweating, and by radiation from the body into the cooler atmosphere. Vasodilation enhances loss of heat through the skin by bringing more blood to the surface of the body. Panting, more common in animals though it does occur in humans, aids heat loss by increasing evaporative heat loss from the moist respiratory tract. At the same time the heat-losing centre depresses the mechanisms that result in heat production, metabolism is slowed down, and muscular activity is decreased.

Variations in thermoregulation. The mechanisms of thermoregulation have been outlined briefly, but a number of factors influence the process of thermoregulation and also the individual's ability to assist with controlling body temperature.

Food intake. Body heat is generated by the metabolism of food, and the body's metabolic rate is increased directly as a result of ingestion of food. This is particularly so when the food eaten is high in protein, and the stimulatory effect may last for as long as 6 hours.

Social drugs. Caffeine increases the metabolic rate, although how it does so is not fully understood. Smoking cigarettes has a similar effect since nicotine stimulates the sympathetic nervous system. Alcohol can increase cooling because it causes vasodilation of the blood vessels in the skin, resulting in a greater loss of heat from the body surface.

Exercise. Body heat is produced by skeletal movement and so the body temperature is related to a person's activity level. The body temperature is highest during periods of great activity and lowest during periods of sleep. Exercise, if overdone, can cause overheating, and exertion-induced heat illness is now a recognized disorder that occurs in basically healthy individuals during or following prolonged strenuous exercise. Heat cramps, heat exhaustion and heat stroke are now not uncommon occurrences at events such as fun-runs, marathons and athletic meetings, and, given the potential danger of severe overheating, caution should be observed and proper precautions taken.

Emotion. Extremes of emotion sometimes affect the body's metabolic rate causing a slight increase in body temperature. Excitement, excessive anxiety or anger may cause an increase in temperature and, indeed, this fact is reflected in such phrases as 'flushed with excitement' and 'hot with rage'. On the other hand, apathy or depression may cause the body temperature to fall.

Hormone levels. Examples are the temperature variations that occur during the female fertility cycle due to the influences of the female sex hormones. Excess production of the hormone thyroxine results from overactivity of the thyroid gland; it increases the body's metabolic rate, thus raising the body temperature. Conversely, with an underactive thyroid gland less thyroxin is produced and body temperature is lower than normal.

Sociocultural norms. Customs concerning clothes can be pertinent. Some religions, for example, dictate the wearing of a head cover at all times, regardless of the environmental temperature. Similarly, ceremonial occasions that are part of a certain culture may demand elaborate dress which is uncomfortably hot in summer weather, or conversely cold in winter. Everyone, too, no matter where in the world, is socialized into acceptance of norms regarding the extent to which clothing can be shed in the hottest weather; this varies between countries, and sometimes between the sexes, and is socioculturally determined rather than by the need for comfort and body temperature control.

Economic status. Many of the activities carried out by individuals in relation to the AL of controlling body temperature need money—to buy clothes, bedding and food; to heat a house and prevent loss of heat from it by excluding draughts, installing double glazing and insulating lofts. Inadequate provisions of this kind may mean that a person is vulnerable to the adverse effects of cold; the two most vulnerable groups in terms of the resultant condition of hypothermia are the young and the elderly. Although public and professional awareness of the problem of hypothermia is now widespread, it has taken a long time for the problem to be given the attention it merits.

So, the individual undoubtedly has some influence on the control of body temperature and, indeed, performs certain deliberate activities to avoid discernible variations. Nevertheless, the body's internal adaptation is paramount in the control of body temperature. If this adaptation were not possible, the scope of human activity would be severely limited and the individual would suffer such discomfort from extremes of heat and cold that everyday living would be disrupted and miserable, and health would be constantly threatened.

The AL of mobilizing.

The capacity for movement is a characteristic of all living things and the ability to move the body freely is a necessary and much valued human activity. Everyday communication, for example, which is so vital to social life, is virtually impossible without movement, involving as it does the acts of speaking and listening, with associated eye movements, facial expression and body language.

Likewise, behaviour associated with the activities of breathing, eating, drinking, eliminating, working, playing and so on all involve movement, and, when asleep, the body systems continue their ceaseless activity. Everyday living involves a multitude of complicated body movements in innumerable combinations, many of them internal and unseen, and many of them not at conscious level.

Mobilizing skills. Physical activity is a basic human drive and is important throughout life. It is the capacity for movement that first allows infants to explore themselves and their environment.

If the child's movement is restricted or if they are deprived of opportunities to respond to stimuli in their surroundings not only physical but also psychological growth may be impeded. This capacity to explore the environment is critical and lack or loss of mobility, or reduced mobility, can have a devastating effect on the youngster's image of self, perhaps even affecting the capacity to take their place effectively in society as adults.

The acquisition of basic mobilizing skills, however, is a very complicated and lengthy process. At birth, the nervous system is not sufficiently developed to permit coordinated musculoskeletal movement and, even when the nervous system is in a state of readiness for learning to take place, human infants, when compared to young animals and birds, are relatively slow to adopt independent coordinated movement. Observation of a baby trying to walk will indicate how many failures there are before the baby manages to stand and walk unsupported and, even then, the sense of balance is unpredictable.

As the body systems develop with age, the healthy growing child is constantly adding to mobilizing skills, and good walking, standing and sitting positions should be cultivated. As well as being aesthetically pleasing to the onlooker, they conserve energy when used in a variety of everyday activities at home, at school and at play; indeed, many recreational activities such as gymnastics, dancing and ice-skating encourage good posture.

Ergonomics. A knowledge of the musculoskeletal system and body mechanisms is essential when analysing mobilizing skills which include, for example, contraction and relaxation of muscles; the mechanics of leverage; the importance of gravity. In fact this knowledge and its application are used to acquire effective techniques of mobilizing, and of moving and handling loads without compromising the musculoskeletal system. However, this biologically weighted interpretation of mobilizing and handling, based on knowledge from the physical sciences, is restricted to muscular bulk and contracting power. There are other components to consider. The science of creating a match between people and their activities, the environment in which they find themselves, and the equipment that they operate is called ergonomics. It is a mix of knowledge from human and physical sciences and is applicable to all human activity, but is of particular relevance to the working world. It looks at how things, jobs and environments are matched to people's sizes, strengths, abilities and other human attributes, and is an example of the interrelatedness of the five factors, discussed later, in our model.

The healthy individual's ability for unaided physical mobility is often taken for granted until circumstances intervene that interfere with part of the musculoskeletal system and its associated pathways.

Threats to mobilizing skills. Fractured or diseased bones are threats to musculoskeletal integrity and can interfere with mobilization in many different ways. Joints too may become diseased and so painful that movement is impeded. Should the hips, knees or ankles be affected, walking becomes difficult; when the small joints of the hands are involved there can be interference with many aspects of mobilizing, for example those used in domestic activities, personal cleansing and dressing, and working and playing. Any form of paralysis such as hemiplegia caused by a cerebrovascular accident (CVA), or paraplegia caused by an accident, severely restricts mobilizing. Of course, even someone with perfectly adequate musculoskeletal and nervous systems may have mobilizing difficulties because of, for example, breathlessness or vision defects, such is the relatedness of the ALs.

For those who have a permanent physical impairment that reduces mobility, the aim is to help them enjoy everyday living to the optimum level. If physically impaired from birth, the goal will be the achievement of a lifestyle where they will have the maximum possible mobility. For those who succumb to an immobilizing disease or injury, it may mean adapting to a lifestyle that is less physically active but just as personally fulfilling; the adaptation may be merely temporary or it may need to be a lifelong adjustment.

It is important that, whatever the age group, people who use mobilizing aids should be helped to understand that they are important as individuals and have equal rights with other members of society. The majority of these people are in the community and, if the disability is likely to be permanent, they will seek optimal independent living within the context of their individual ability, not their disability.

Public attitudes to disability. Those who are dependent for mobilizing can be distressed by the public's attitude to their dependence. Some members of the public show their discomfort by using 'distancing' techniques which make disabled people feel uncomfortable; some may be embarrassingly over-solicitous; others manage a mature interaction, conveying that the disabled person is valued as a 'person', yet acknowledging, probably by non-verbal communication, the reality of the dependence. For children who have a disability such as a leg amputation, the child's problem is also the problem of the parents, and the youngster may have to endure harsh teasing from their peer group.

It is desirable that able-bodied people should become more aware of the ways in which such people can be helped to achieve a satisfactory lifestyle in work, leisure, recreation and family situations. Adequate provision for their needs will overcome their disadvantages to some extent and help them to make the positive contribution they are so competent to make in the community where they live. Positive coping strategies can certainly offset an individual's problems with the AL of mobilizing.

The AL of working and playing

Broadly speaking, most people spend about one-third of the day sleeping, and the rest working and playing. Work and play are complementary, and both are fundamental aspects of living. The activities of working and playing have many dimensions and, particularly according to the different stages of the lifespan, their nature and purpose are open to various interpretations.

Working is the word most commonly used to describe an individual's main daily activity and tends to be thought of, firstly, in terms of gainful employment. People work to earn an income in order to provide for the necessities of living for themselves, and for their dependants. Because work is necessary, it is often thought of in a rather negative way, but, in fact, a job not only provides an income, but is also an important part of a person's identity; it provides a sense of purpose and accomplishment; a structure to each day and year; a source of company (although teleworking from home is becoming more common); and a defined status in the family and in society. Those who are unemployed are deprived of these benefits and the right to earn a living. Nevertheless they—like others such as students, homemakers, voluntary workers and retired people—would still describe much of their daily activity as 'work'. So, although discussion of the nature of the activity of 'working' inevitably focuses on gainful employment, the broader interpretation of the term should not be forgotten.`

Even when work is for financial gain, remuneration is not the only consideration when choosing a job or career. For example, teaching or nursing or medicine are frequently chosen by those who wish 'to work with people'. Others pursue their jobs as an opportunity to use their hands or their intellect, or to use particular qualifications, to be able to travel, or to gain power. People who choose to do voluntary work see their purpose as giving service to the community. Adults who stay at home to look after children would describe their purpose in terms of their children's well-being, and it is noteworthy that in a number of industrialized countries there is a changing or merging of the male and female roles in that it may be the mother who is in paid employment and the father or partner who is at home caring for the children. However, whatever the job, be it paid or unpaid, prevention of boredom and meaningful use of time are basic reasons for working.

Playing is the term being used to describe what a person does in 'non-work' time. It infers that 'playing' is the opposite of 'working', and in the context of this model it is an all-inclusive term that covers many other terms such as leisure, relaxation, recreation, hobby, exercise, sport, holiday. As unemployment has grown in some communities, retirement is earlier and working hours are shorter, and there has been increased interest in the use of leisure. Enjoyment and occupation of time are prime objectives in all forms of playing, and for children it is also a means of learning and developing.

Health and safety at work. Promoting health at work is good business sense and nowadays, in many countries, there are stringent government regulations about health and safety at work. These link with the AL of maintaining a safe environment: protective clothing; guarded machinery; control of noise, temperature and lighting levels; legal requirements about moving and handling loads, and about handling hazardous substances; and provision of ergonomically friendly workstations.

Apart from physical safety, there is the potentially harmful risk of working in a setting that is too demanding emotionally. Excessive stress may be caused by the pressure of work, and extremely long working hours have become increasingly common, particularly in the UK. However, even when working within normal hours, stress may be caused by workplace problems, or by concern about work commitments clashing with family/home responsibilities. Increasingly, both employers and governments are accepting that there is a need to introduce family-friendly workplace policies such as flexitime hours and the availability of childcare facilities. Of course, personal coping strategies, peer group support, counselling and education can also contribute to the alleviation of stress. Learning to 'manage stress' is immediately important when it has adverse effects, but the long-term strategy is to deal with the cause.

The rate of change in current technology may, in fact, cause some of the stress at work. Acquired skills can rapidly become outdated and necessitate training for a second or third type of employment in a lifetime; indeed, some of the technological advances involve replacing people with machines. The resulting unemployment is a crucial politicoeconomic issue in much of the industrialized world.

Unemployment and retirement. Unemployment is known to cause considerable psychological distress to the individual and to the family. Not only is there loss of financial independence, but also the loss of self-esteem and self-confidence; there are humiliating experiences when job applications are rejected; there is a decline in social standing; and a loss of social contacts. These losses can lead to feelings of frustration and anger, or to depression and a feeling of worthlessness, even to the point of contemplating suicide.

Although different from unemployment, retirement from work does sometimes cause reactions that are similar to the 'worthlessness' of unemployment. The syndrome is now well recognized, to the extent that pre- and post-retirement courses are planned to help people disengage from work and to re-engage in leisure.

Capacity for leisure. Although in relative terms more people nowadays have more time for leisure and more money, many recreational pursuits are expensive and this can be a problem for the lowest paid workers, parents with several children, lone parents, students, the unemployed and pensioners. In some countries, this fact is recognized and they may be offered, for example, reduced rates for travelling or for entrance to leisure activities. There is no doubt that, with less work, there will be greater emphasis on play. Education for leisure and the provision of affordable recreational facilities will therefore assume even greater political importance in the future.

However, in some developing countries there is no question of seeking leisure; even the children cannot indulge in play. A number of countries in southern Asia are reputed to use millions of child labourers, many of them in bondage, for example in gem-cutting, pottery, mining and the carpet industry. Theoretically, a battery of laws protects them from exploitation and various welfare groups cooperate to oppose such child slavery, but these measures have limited impact. Such children will never know school or the luxury of playing, but their family's survival often depends on the meagre sum they earn from working.

The AL of expressing sexuality

'It's a boy' or 'It's a girl' is almost always the first announcement on delivery of a newborn baby, if indeed parents have not been told the sex during an ultrasonographic examination in pregnancy. As the basic body structure of males and females is distinctly different even at birth, identification of the baby's sex is almost instantaneous and, throughout the entire lifespan, sexuality is a significant dimension of personality and interpersonal behaviour.

Each human being is a 'sexual' human being and has a sexual identity; that is, there is a perception of 'self' as a boy or a girl, then as a man or a woman. The ways in which sexuality is expressed vary according to culture but, in any given society, males and females tend to show differentiation in a variety of ways other than those determined simply by biological difference. Invariably, men and women adopt different styles of dress; traditionally, males and females have tended to occupy different roles, both domestically and socially, although in many parts of the world long-established differences between the sexes are fast disappearing. Currently there is a more egalitarian view of the roles of men and women and, at the same time, social mores have become more liberal in terms of the ways in which sexuality is expressed. There is less rigid interpretation of activities, attitudes, beliefs and values associated with expressing sexuality as being 'good' or 'bad', 'normal' or 'abnormal'. The subject of sex is no longer taboo: it is aired by the media and discussed in school and at home and, as a result, people are becoming more aware of the many dimensions of the AL of expressing sexuality, not least in terms of its relationship to health and illness.

Sociocultural similarities and differences. Individuals learn to adopt the norms and morals of their society through the process of socialization. Parents influence the child's sexual development from an early age; femininity or masculinity can be encouraged by the particular choice of clothes and games, and by the sexual behaviour of the parents themselves. Nowadays, because of varied forms of 'family' (i.e. more lone parent families, more step families, and more children reared by couples of the same sex) and through exposure to more liberal media, children must be growing up with a more realistic view of the variety in adult relationships. School education further shapes the child's developing concept of sexuality, and gradually each individual begins to learn society's expectations of how men and women may behave, and how sexuality may be expressed, both privately and publicly.

While forms of sexual expression vary considerably from one society to another, similar forms of behaviour to attract a sexual partner are universal. Physical appearance is of considerable importance in this, although there are no uniform standards of sexual attractiveness.

Social permissiveness. While universal regulations prohibit some particularly undesirable sexual relationships such as incest and adult sexual intercourse with children, most societies have their own laws delineating the forms of sexual partnerships that are acceptable. In Western civilization the monogamous marriage (or long-term partnership) is still the norm but there is almost more variety than uniformity as a result of the so-called 'sexual revolution' of the latter decades of the twentieth century.

Social permissiveness has brought many benefits but also some problems. Never before has Western society had such large numbers of people stressed by dissatisfaction about sexual inadequacy; marital disharmony; difficulties of separation and divorce; the strains of lone parenting; and the distress of sexual abuse in the form of incest, rape and sexual assault. The growing invasion of pornography, especially through the Internet, is another unsavoury trend in relation to the potential harm to children.

Social permissiveness towards sex has removed the stigma that used to be attached to multiple sexual partnerships; such behaviour, made more possible by more widely available and reliable contraception and by frequent travel around the world, has resulted in the ever-increasing problem of sexually transmitted disease (STD). Although this is by no means a new problem for society, it was highlighted as a result of the acquired immune deficiency syndrome (AIDS) epidemic which in the 1980s became recognized as a major health threat throughout the world. The virus responsible for AIDS was isolated in 1983 and named the human immunodeficiency virus (HIV). Not everyone with HIV infection develops AIDS but, for those who do, there is still no cure or vaccine, and preventing the further spread of HIV infection is therefore vital. Public education is the main means of prevention. Safe sex (especially by the use of condoms) and a reduction in the rate of partner exchange are the main goals. According to world figures produced by UNAIDS, the United Nations AIDS Agency, and the WHO in 1998, there were 30.6 million people living with AIDS and an estimated 16 000 new HIV infections per day.

Sexual orientation. Undoubtedly modes of sexual behaviour are shaped as well as restricted by social pressure. Preference for *heterosexuality* is still the norm for the majority of adults, but sexual attraction to a person of the same sex (*homosexuality*) has existed through the ages and is found in all societies. In Western countries today, there is greater enlightenment, and acceptance of the right of consenting adults, to choose a homosexual relationship. Of course, some homosexuals are also heterosexual (i.e. *bisexual*) and may marry and have children; homosexuality is not an absolute state but a sexual orientation on a continuum that ranges from exclusively heterosexual to exclusively homosexual.

There are a few people who, even in childhood, feel that they have been born into the sex opposite to their actual body structure. *Transsexualism* has as its central feature altered gender identity, and the transsexual not only dresses and acts like a person of the opposite sex, but usually wants to have surgery and treatment to make the body like that of the opposite sex, although this may not be possible. *Transvestites*, on the other hand, although they dress in clothes of the opposite sex for sexual gratification, do not generally wish to belong to the opposite sex.

So, there is considerable variation, and individuals are now much more prepared to declare, publicly, their sexual orientation.

Pregnancy, childbirth and fertility. Obviously there are many aspects to the AL of expressing sexuality but sexual intercourse is an important component of adult relationships—and essential for the continuation of the species. So sexual intercourse, pregnancy and childbirth are of enormous significance for the couple involved in personal terms, as well as socially and economically.

Along with the physical changes that occur in the mother's body, pregnancy is also a time of emotional adaptation. Increasingly, prenatal education and support is taking account of this fact and includes the emotional preparation of the woman and her partner for the birth and postnatal period. Appreciation of the need for this type of support is reflected in the positive encouragement that is now given for partners to be involved in prenatal classes and to be present at the birth.

In contradistinction, some pregnancies are unwanted. In an attempt to reduce their incidence, contraceptive protection is widely advocated, quite publicly, and in many countries contraceptive devices are subsidized or even provided free of charge. In fact, the ever-increasing world population has to be regarded as one of the major economic issues for the twenty-first century, quite apart from the personal distress of many of the unwanted children.

In recent years, of course, advances in reproductive technology have made possible in vitro fertilization and even 'posthumous conception'. And currently, the possibility of cloning human beings provokes heated controversy about the potential use or abuse of such powerful knowledge, not to mention the related legal and ethical issues.

The AL of expressing sexuality is a vast and complex dimension of living.

The AL of sleeping

All parents are familiar with their children asking, 'Why do we have to go to bed?'. Most parents believe that because children are growing, they need relatively more sleep than adults and, indeed, there is scientific evidence to support this idea. Adults vary more in the amount of sleep they require but, on average, spend about one-quarter to one-third of their lives sleeping. In terms of time alone then, sleeping is for everyone an important AL.

To include sleeping as an 'activity' is not paradoxical, for, although sleep provides the greatest degree of rest, the body systems are still functioning albeit at a reduced level. Sleep has been described as a recurrent state of inertia and unresponsiveness, a state in which a person does not respond overtly to what is going on in the surrounding environment. Although consciousness is lost temporarily, a sufficient new stimulus, such as an alarm clock going off, will rouse the person. So sleeping is quite different from the states of coma and anaesthesia.

Most people sleep with closed eyes; they lie still for part of the time, but they move at intervals throughout the sleep periods; sometimes there is relaxation in the muscles of the face and neck so that the jaw is unsupported and the mouth open; breathing is slower and usually deeper; flaccid muscles in the upper respiratory tract are thought to be responsible for snoring. But what is the nature of this phenomenon called sleep?

For many years, this very question has been exercising experts in various parts of the world, and the information that has accumulated from sleep research has been vital to understanding the nature and function of sleep.

The sleep cycle. Each sleep cycle is approximately 90–100 minutes in duration and there are usually four to six cycles in a person's normal sleep period, each described as having five stages. The first four stages are what is described as non-rapid eye movement sleep (NREM) and the fifth is REM sleep. Characteristics of the stages of sleep are described in Box 2.3 and a sleep cycle in Figure. 2.5.

There is a cycle of NREM and REM sleep throughout the night. A baby's sleep has more REM than NREM stages; with increasing age, there is less REM sleep. If awakened during the REM stages, people may report vivid dreams, and it is thought that dreams may promote psychological integration. Since REM sleep also occurs in the fetus, its function may be described more simply as organizing electrical circuits within the brain.

Although everyone's sleep has cycles, there is considerable variation in the length of time that people spend sleeping, and in what is considered 'sufficient' sleep.

Psychological aspects. So, sleeping is influenced by a variety of biological factors and, in turn, sleep–wake rhythms affect the physiology and biochemistry of the human body, but the individual's psychological status is linked to sleeping in a number of ways.

As an example of extremes, mood can be considered as a continuum with excitement at one pole and depression at the other.

Box 2.3   Stages of sleep

Stage 1
This is the transition from wakefulness to sleep. The sleeper has just 'dropped off'. There is a general relaxation; there are fleeting thoughts, and the sleeper can be wakened by any slight stimulus. If awakened, the stage is remembered merely as one of drowsiness; it is not described as sleep. But, if not interrupted, the next stage is entered after about 15 minutes.

Stage 2
There is greater relaxation, and thoughts have a dream-like quality. The sleeper is unmistakedly asleep but can be wakened easily.

Stage 3
This stage usually occurs after 30 minutes of sleep. There is complete relaxation and the pulse rate slows, as do most other bodily functions. Familiar noises such as a flushing toilet do not usually waken the sleeper. If undisturbed, the next stage follows.

Stage 4
The sleeper is relaxed, rarely moves, is difficult to waken, and is in a 'deep sleep'. If sleep-walking occurs, or if there is enuresis, it occurs at this stage. (Stages 3 and 4 collectively are known as 'slow wave sleep' because, on an electroencephalograph, they show as low frequency, synchronized waves.)

Stage 5
This is the stage of sleep during which most dreaming occurs. The eyes move rapidly back and forth giving the name rapid eye movement (REM) sleep to this stage. Physiologically, REM sleep is remarkably similar to wakefulness.

Transient insomnia caused by excitement has been experienced by most people and may not cause undue distress. The sleeplessness associated with depression may, however, be severe, and may continue over time. The depressed person can lie awake for hours dwelling on unhappy themes of hopelessness and, when sleep does come, is easily wakened, only to resume thoughts of rejection and failure, or even suicide. The primary characteristic of sleep change in depression is early morning wakening; indeed, it is a major diagnostic feature.

Whatever the 'science' of sleep, and whatever the quantity or quality of sleep, the psychological effect of wakening up refreshed or unrefreshed determines a person's belief about being a good or bad sleeper; in other words, assessment of sleep is largely subjective.

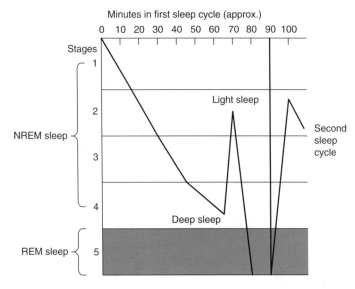

Figure 2.5 A sleep cycle.

Environmental aspects. Sleep can be affected by a number of environmental factors. Sleep tends to come more easily in a familiar environment—a cool, quiet, dark room in surroundings which are well known, with personal belongings at hand and so on, although this may vary according to cultural norms. In Western cultures, it is usual for a cohabiting couple to sleep together in one bed, but most other people sleep alone. However, in some cultures, it is not uncommon for several members of the family to sleep together in the same 'sleeping' space.

Environmental noise may or may not affect sleep. Again, familiarity with the environment allows many people to sleep despite, for example, the noise of a busy thoroughfare or an aircraft flight path. Night-shift workers may have major complaints about noise when they are attempting to sleep during the day, although, if habitually on night shift, many seem to learn to ignore background noise.

Environmental temperature may affect the ability to fall asleep and to remain asleep. The body temperature falls during sleep, and a further lowering of room temperature usually wakens the sleeper, as indeed does any increase.

Perhaps to be expected, the climate has an influence, and where there are extremes of climate attempts are made to control and modify the indoor temperature. In hot climates, bedrooms increasingly are equipped with air-conditioning systems; in cold climates, insulation and central heating systems provide heat and warmth. Being without a home can, of course, cause problems. In the UK, as in many other countries, the number of homeless people has increased in recent times. For the homeless, sleeping 'rough', exposed to unfavourable weather conditions which endanger health, is certainly not conducive to satisfactory sleep.

To many people, sleeping is taken for granted, but there are many circumstances that can affect a person's ability to benefit from the AL of sleeping.

The AL of dying

Dying is the final act of living. To die suddenly from natural causes in old age, and without loss of dignity, is what most people would regard as a 'good death'. However, death is often preceded by a period of survival in a state of terminal illness, the duration of which may be prolonged, and perhaps accompanied by pain and distress. It is in these circumstances that the issue of euthanasia is sometimes raised.

Euthanasia and 'living wills'. 'Bringing about an easy death' is the actual meaning of the term euthanasia, although 'mercy killing' is a phrase often used as a synonym. It is a topic that evokes strong emotions and heated debate. Those with particular religious or personal convictions argue that it is morally wrong to end life deliberately (active euthanasia). Others consider that euthanasia need not be a deliberate act of killing but merely allows death to occur, for example by withholding antibiotics at the onset of a respiratory infection in an old, incapacitated person although providing care and comfort in every other way (passive euthanasia).

In a number of countries proponents of euthanasia have formed societies—the first was in the UK in 1935—to discuss and propagate their beliefs and to provide information to people who wish assistance in reducing the distress of dying. In some instances, an even more positive stance has been taken and attempts have been made to introduce legislation making voluntary euthanasia permissible.

In relation to any consideration of euthanasia, patient autonomy is obviously a crucial issue and in the last few decades, although not binding in law, there has been increasing interest in the concept of the 'living will'. It is a type of advance directive signed when the person is in full possession of all their faculties; in essence, it indicates that they do not wish to be involved in life-prolonging treatment and that healthcare staff should take account of their wishes.

The euthanasia debate is not new and history records examples of group euthanasia practices in Greece in the first century BC. It has gone on down the centuries but the debate is certainly rekindled by technological advances where complex life support systems are available for patients who, previously, could not have survived.

Accident, violence and suicide. In contrast to death from natural causes, some people die as a result of accident, violence or suicide.

Accidental death. In most countries of the Western world, accidents, notably road accidents, are a major cause of death in children and young adults. Other types of accident may cause mass death: international publicity is given to serious aircraft accidents which, although rare, almost always have a high mortality rate; industrial accidents, for example in mines, often cause mass deaths in large numbers; and in areas of the world where natural disasters such as floods, earthquakes and hurricanes occur with relative frequency, there may be a heavy death toll. Every country has its major tragedies when whole families or even communities can be wiped out by such events.

Violent death. Sudden violent death may not be accidental, but deliberate. Murder is not common but the incidence is rising in most industrialized nations. Most countries are aware of the increasing violence and terrorism in the modern world and of the corresponding need to protect individuals from undesirable and preventable acts of homicide. For many obvious reasons, relatives' grief may be complicated by feelings of lust for revenge and fear for their own personal safety, and such circumstances may precipitate yet more deaths.

Violent death on a large scale as a result of war seems to be a continuing feature in modern society. Following the Second World War, the United Nations Organization was created to provide a forum for discussion about disputes in order to preclude the waging of war. Unfortunately, as evident in recent history, there can be failure to reach negotiated settlements and the death toll among civilians and armed forces continues in countries still at war.

The possibility of a nuclear holocaust and the prospect of mass annihilation loomed large in the era of the 'cold war'. Although the nuclear threat has lessened, there is still need for efforts at international level to ensure that it will never return.

Suicide. There are some individuals who, for a variety of reasons, want to die and intentionally take their own lives by committing suicide. Suicide is no longer a crime in most countries, including the UK, but there is still a stigma attached to suicide, and this may serve to increase the already great amount of distress and guilt suffered by the relatives.

Emotional aspects. It has to be acknowledged that, for most people, death is accompanied by intense fear. Insight into people's feelings about dying was first provided by the in-depth research interviews with dying patients which Kübler-Ross conducted and analysed as long ago as 1969. She described how most people pass through a phase of 'denial and isolation' in which they refuse to accept that they are dying. As denial lessens, the common reaction is one of 'anger', then attempts to cope with the situation sometimes involve a stage of 'bargaining'. The person tries to find ways of believing that a miracle recovery will happen or that they might make 'bargains' with the doctor or with God. When these fail and the imminent loss of life and loved ones becomes a reality, 'depression' is experienced and this is an almost universal feature of the dying process. There is profound regret over missed opportunities and failures of the past and an overwhelming sadness engulfs the dying person. It should be realized, however, that these phases are not necessarily a linear progression: there is overlap and movement back and forth and, in any case, each person has a unique way of dealing with these powerful emotions.

Beliefs and customs. Most people have some kind of personal belief about the meaning of death and often this is based on the philosophy of a particular religion. Most religions have some strong belief about the fate of the human spirit and soul after death. For example, Christianity purports that there is life after death, that this existence is everlasting and will hold greater joy and peace than life on earth.

For those who do not hold religious beliefs, dying may be seen to have no purpose other than to bring an inevitable end to living;

a coming to terms with the finiteness of life. And perhaps, albeit subconsciously, some of the grieving in bereavement is a form of grief for oneself; another's death is a reminder of one's own death, a reminder of the transience of life and the fact that the lifespan is not never ending.

Each society has its own way of treating death according to its culture. In societies where care of the dying is still very much a family responsibility, the social customs that surround death tend to be elaborate and are designed to encourage the bereaved to mourn openly and to seek the sympathy and support of members of their community. Many of the social customs surrounding death have their origin in religion and involve a ceremonial that ensures proper disposal of the dead body, for example when the person is a Muslim, Hindu or orthodox Jew. But in Western societies elaborate ritual surrounding death is fast disappearing and the occasion of the funeral is often used to 'celebrate the person's life' rather than mourn the death.

It is difficult to reflect on the nature of death and dying without considering the nature of grieving and bereavement. Most adults have some experience of these emotions following the death of a relative or friend; indeed grieving and bereavement are a part of the process of living, although related to the process of dying and death.

Grief and bereavement. Following the death of someone significant to them, those who are left behind almost inevitably suffer a deep sense of desolation. It is not necessarily only husbands, wives or children who are bereaved, although one's immediate reaction is to think of these close relatives. So intense is the emotion of grief that it affects even those sometimes wrongly assumed to be untouched by loss: the very young and the very old, the mentally ill and the mentally disabled. 'The bereaved' are, by definition, those who suffer loss and grieve in response to a death, those who were, in some important way, committed to the person who died—it is the 'cost of commitment'.

Although feelings of loss and grief are almost universal responses in bereavement, many other reactions can occur. Shock, disbelief, anger, denial, shame, guilt, resentment, anxiety, fear, depression and despair are among the emotional reactions that may be experienced by the bereaved to a varying degree and at different times throughout the grieving process. Even long after the death, episodes of intense grief and despair may return.

Bereavement can be a long, painful and lonely process. Although it is probably true that time heals, a person seldom remains unaffected by a bereavement even after a long time lapse. It is not that they forget the dead person, but perhaps time gives them practice in adapting to living in changed circumstances.

Even from such a brief description of the 12 ALs, it is clear that conceptualizing 'living' as an amalgam of 'activities' is a helpful way of beginning to think simply yet constructively about the complex process of living. All of the ALs are important, although obviously some have greater priority than others; the AL of breathing is of prime importance. However, the order in which the ALs are listed does not reflect an order of priority because, according to circumstances, a person's priorities change. Also, as previously mentioned, although the 12 ALs are described separately, they are very closely related to one another. Indeed, although the ALs are presented as one concept of the model, they should not be thought of in isolation since they are affected by the other components and these too are closely related to one another. Nevertheless, in their own right, each of the concepts contributes another dimension of 'living', as the following discussion will show.

Lifespan

It is easy to appreciate why the concept of lifespan is included as one component of the model of living: 'living' is concerned with the whole of a person's life. Each person has a lifespan from birth to death, and stage on the lifespan—infancy, childhood, adolescence, adulthood, senior citizenship—influences the individual's behaviour for each AL. These stages are mentioned in more detail in the model of nursing.

The lifespan is represented in the diagram of the model of living by a line, arrowed to indicate the unidirectional movement from birth to death (Fig. 2.6). Of course, all people do not live through all stages of the lifespan; some die at birth, and some otherwise healthy people die prematurely, for example as a result of accident or disease. So, although each person has a lifespan from birth to death, its length is variable.

Most countries have local registry offices where, as a legal requirement, births and deaths are recorded, and it is from these

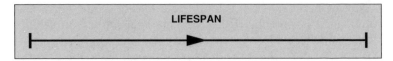

Figure 2.6 The lifespan.

data that local and national birth and death rates are calculated. The collection of statistics about birth and death, and causes of death, provides a general picture of the health of a population. For example, using these statistics the life expectancy of a given population can be predicted; infant mortality rates can be used as an audit index when comparing health services in different countries; and the age range of people dying from particular diseases or road traffic accidents can guide the activities of health education programmes and related prevention procedures.

These data are also valuable in relation to the provision of a national education system. In most countries there is a statutory age for entering, and a minimum age for leaving, school, so data about the population give guidance about the number and location of state schools, and to some extent the provision that is made for establishments associated with higher education.

Such data about the lifespan are also used in relation to employment, and thus eligibility for a state retirement pension. And, of course, people who are unemployed, for whatever reason, come under the protective umbrella of the social services in such countries. In relation to work opportunities, there is currently concern about ageism—discrimination on grounds of advancing age. It can occur even as young as the 30s age group, for example when seeking employment following redundancy from a previous job. It may be that this is an economic issue in that an employer usually pays a lower salary to younger, less experienced staff. Or it may be a skills issue: in a fast-changing technological era, skills quickly become outdated and frequent updating—or indeed training in new or different skills—is demanded by employers. In fact, the age of retirement, as such, can be blurred by the age of redundancy and unemployment.

So these data collected centrally at the Office of National Statistics (or equivalent), indicating the age structure of a population, have applications within the structure of government that affect many aspects of everyday living, not least of which is taxation: the number of people at work and paying taxes as against the number of dependent children; the number unemployed and dependent; and the number on retirement pensions.

Inevitably, as a person moves along the lifespan, there is continuous change and every aspect of living is influenced by the biological, psychological, sociocultural, environmental and politicoeconomic circumstances encountered. Inevitably, too, at different stages of the lifespan there are varying degrees of dependence and independence in the activities of living.

Dependence/independence continuum

This concept of the model is closely related to the lifespan and to the ALs. It is included to acknowledge that there are stages of the lifespan when a person cannot yet (or for various reasons, can no longer) perform certain ALs independently. Each person could be said to have a *dependence/independence continuum* for each AL. As shown below (Fig. 2.7), the terms 'total dependence' and 'total independence' are used to describe the poles of the continuum and the arrows indicate that movement can take place in either direction according to circumstances. We define independence as 'ability to achieve the AL to a personally and socially acceptable standard without help'.

To emphasize that the dependence/independence continuum relates to each of the ALs—when referring it to the person as a whole the concept is too global to be meaningful—the continuum appears in the diagrammatic representation of the model of living alongside each of the 12 activities (Fig. 2.8).

A person's position could be plotted on each continuum (at either pole or somewhere between) to provide an impression of the degree of dependence or independence in respect of the 12 ALs. If repeated at intervals of time, any obvious change in direction or movement along the continua would become apparent.

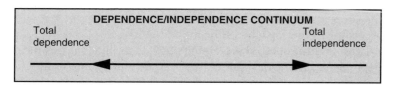

Figure 2.7   The dependence/independence continuum.

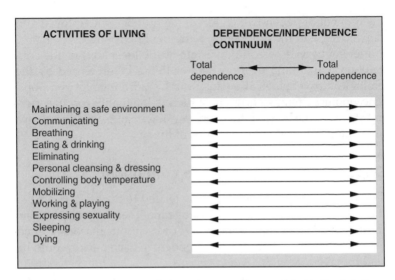

Figure 2.8 The dependence/independence continuum related to the Activities of Living.

Comparison of the dependence/independence status of people at different stages of the lifespan illustrates the close links between these two concepts of the model. Newborn babies are dependent on others for help with most of the ALs. From this state of almost total dependence, each child according to capacity can be visualized as gradually moving along the continuum towards the independent pole for each AL.

From collected data there are statistical averages for the age at which independence is achieved for particular ALs. However, there are always exceptions; by no means everyone has the capacity or opportunity to achieve or retain independence in all of the ALs. Not all children are born with the potential for 'total independence', whether as a result of severe physical or learning disability, or both. In such circumstances, progress during infancy and childhood cannot be measured against normal development milestones and the goal is maximum independence in the ALs according to the capacity of the individual child.

Even in adulthood, there are circumstances that can result in dependence in one or more of the ALs: obvious examples are illness and accident. Dependence may be on help from other people or on special aids and equipment, for example a wheelchair that provides '*aided independence*' for the AL of mobilizing. Indeed, in a broader context, even healthy able-bodied adults are dependent on others for their so-called 'independence' in many of the ALs; for example, in much of the developed world, for the AL of eating and drinking there is dependence on people such as the farmer, fisherman, factory worker and shopkeeper, and on various types of equipment and a supply of safe water and heat which aid preparation and cooking of food and drink.

There is, therefore, no absolute state of 'independence' in the ALs. The concepts of 'dependence' and 'independence' are really meaningful only when considered as relative to one another, hence the reason for presenting these ideas in our model of living by means of a dependence/independence *continuum*. Change in dependence/independence status for one AL can, because the ALs are so closely related, cause change in status for one or more of the others.

The dependence/independence status of an individual in relation to ALs is not linked only to lifespan: it is also closely associated with the factors that influence ALs.

Factors influencing the ALs

So far, three concepts of the model have been described: the ALs, the lifespan, and the dependence/independence continuum. However, although everyone carries out ALs (at whatever stage of the lifespan and with varying degrees of independence), each individual does so differently. To a large extent these differences arise because a variety of factors have influenced or are influencing the way a person carries out ALs, and these 'factors' form the fourth concept of the model.

It would be possible to devise a long list of the different factors: for example, biological, intellectual, emotional, social, cultural, spiritual, religious, ethical, philosophical, environmental, political, economic and legal factors. However, one of the intentions when creating a model is that it should not *seem* excessively complicated, so the factors influencing the ALs are described in five main groups: biological, psychological, sociocultural, environmental, and politicoeconomic factors (Fig. 2.9). It must be noted, however, that intellectual and emotional factors are subsumed under psychological factors; that spiritual, religious, philosophical and ethical factors are subsumed under sociocultural factors,

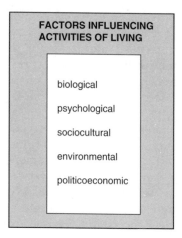

FACTORS INFLUENCING ACTIVITIES OF LIVING

biological

psychological

sociocultural

environmental

politicoeconomic

Figure 2.9 The factors influencing the Activities of Living.

because for this model of living it is considered that such values and beliefs often find expression within a particular cultural view; and that legal factors are subsumed under politicoeconomic factors.

The factors are deliberately focused on the ALs. It would be possible to focus them on the individual as a total entity discussing in general terms the effects of the five groups of factors on lifestyle, but this is too global. In preference, discussing them as they influence each of the 12 ALs highlights the individuality in different manifestations of living.

The factors, the ALs, the lifespan and the dependence/independence continuum are interlinked, and the five factors themselves are interlinked. Each factor involves a huge area of human knowledge and students will have specific textbooks and study related to these topics in other parts of the curriculum. At this stage, however, for the purposes of discussion, a few general points will be made about each factor separately.

Biological

For the purposes of this model of living, the term biological relates to the human body's anatomical and physiological performance. This is partly determined by the individual's genetic inheritance. In recent years, there have been spectacular advances in the science of genetics and the current Human Genome Project involves international collaboration on research to map out the entire genetic blueprint (genome) of the human being. Among other things it can, for example:

- give scientists a complete molecular understanding of human beings
- assist an understanding of what goes wrong when disease interferes with normal functioning
- provide pharmaceutical companies with new therapeutic targets.

Of course, in the process of studying human genetic variations and susceptibility to disease, there is enormous potential for abuse of this powerful knowledge; there are innumerable ethical, legal and social implications. Although the influence of genetic inheritance is usually more obvious in facial appearance and physique, it also affects each person's overall physical performance. The individual's physical endowment is important in its own right, but it is inextricably linked with other factors—psychological, sociocultural, environmental and politicoeconomic.

Not only are the biological factors interlinked with these others: as a group, the factors are related to the other components of the model. Even in a healthy person, for example, the body's physical ability varies according to age (i.e. the lifespan component of the model), and influences the degree of independence possible to the individual (i.e. the dependence/independence continuum), so inevitably the factors influence the person's individuality in living and affect the way each person carries out the ALs. Despite the phenomenal physical growth of the fetus in utero, a newborn baby is far from biological maturity and, unlike most animals, there are many years of further growth before reaching the physical competence and independence synonymous with young adulthood in the human. At the other end of the lifespan, the physical ability of the older person is gradually less efficient and there may be an insidious loss of independence. It is logical to expect, therefore, that the biological state of the body has an important contributing influence on the individual's ALs throughout the lifespan. However, it must be emphasized that it is only for the purposes of discussion that biological factors are singled out; it is the overall consideration of the person that is important, and other factors are involved.

Psychological

Psychological factors cannot be considered in isolation; they are related to biological and also to sociocultural, environmental and politicoeconomic factors. As well as being related to the other four factors, psychological factors are related to the other components of the model. They influence living throughout the lifespan, especially intellectual and emotional development, and have a bearing on the person's level of independence; so inevitably they influence the person's individuality in living, and affect the way each person carries out the ALs.

Intellectual aspects. The term 'cognitive development' is often used to refer to the process of acquiring intellectual skills—thinking, reasoning and problem-solving—which are essential for physical survival and affect all ALs. The process by which people obtain information about themselves and their environment begins as a baby. Via the sense organs, the baby perceives stimuli such as pressure, pain, warmth, cold, taste, sound, changes in light intensity and various visual images. At first, the response to many of these stimuli may be simply a reflex action, because highly differentiated responses are not possible until the cerebral cortex grows and conceptual processes begin to develop.

It is important to remember that sensory deprivation, for example visual or hearing impairment, may result in delayed intellectual development and that this can affect almost every AL. It is just as important to remember that lack of stimulation during the early years of life at home and at school can retard intellectual development. Indeed the neglected child, even with a genetic inheritance which would promise high potential, has less opportunity to develop intellectually and emotionally, thereby affecting ALs such as maintaining a safe environment, communicating, and working and playing.

Intellectual development continues in childhood and early adolescence by means of formal education and the pursuit of personal interests and leisure. In late adolescence, there is usually a more marked differentiation between individuals, and this can affect decisions about advanced studies and choice of job or career. Establishment in an occupation is one of the major tasks during adulthood and the significance of the AL of working and playing is paramount.

During the ageing process, overall intellectual functioning becomes gradually less efficient and may cause problems with ALs; for example, there may be difficulty with communication because the senses are less acute; maintaining a safe environment in the home may be less easy as memory fails; opportunities for fulfilling the AL of working and playing may be reduced, and boredom or loneliness may result. However, an enhancing environment can help to sustain even an elderly person's intellectual status, making it possible to remain independent for the majority of ALs, thus facilitating residence in the community rather than resorting to care in an institutional setting.

Emotional aspects. Like intellectual development, emotional development is closely related to lifespan and the growth of independence in the relevant ALs. The need for love and belonging is crucial in young children; and from a stable and close relationship in infancy, the child can grow with self-confidence, develop self-esteem and acquire a positive self-image. The development of personality is one of the outcomes of emotional development. Early sex-related behaviour patterns tend to be strengthened and the child often models on the parent of the same sex, sometimes through the AL of playing. Parents or parent substitutes are significant in influencing emotional development, and the acquisition of norms and moral standards is part of communicating in the model of living.

Emotional development during the teens is closely related to the biological changes of puberty. Emotional relationships with parents undergo change and adolescents begin to assert their individuality and independence, at first for the 'playing' part of the AL of working and playing, and eventually for working; they may resist adult authority and advice.

During young adulthood, there are usually important emotional relationships associated with courtship and setting up house with a partner (usually of the opposite sex) and the rearing of children, all associated with the AL of expressing sexuality. Consequently late adulthood may bring with it major emotional readjustments when grown-up children leave home; there may often be an experience of tremendous loss, although there may also be a new sense of freedom to enjoy the 'playing' part of the AL of working and playing.

For the older person there may have to be many emotional adaptations related to the physical effects of ageing and sometimes declining intellectual ability which can influence ALs such as maintaining a safe environment, communicating and expressing sexuality. There are reduced opportunities for emotional and social relationships as family and friends in their peer group die, which influences the bereavement and grieving part of the AL of dying in the model.

There are individual differences. There are marked variations in the capacity for intellectual development, and enormous differences related to the general ability to cope with the emotional demands of life events. And, of course, this intellectual and emotional development takes place not only within the family: it also develops in the context of the society and culture in which the individual lives.

Sociocultural

For the purposes of the model of living, the term sociocultural subsumes spiritual, religious and ethical aspects of living. As well as being related to the other four factors, sociocultural factors are related to the other components of the model. They influence living throughout the lifespan and have a bearing on the person's level of independence, so inevitably they influence the person's individuality in living and affect the way each person carries out the ALs. Out of a vast range of knowledge in the disciplines associated with the social sciences, a few concepts have been selected to illustrate their relevance to 'living' and the model of living.

Culture. Within every society there is some kind of organization of people into groups and of activities into institutions. The social organization may be simple, as in a nomadic tribe, or it may involve a highly elaborate network of groups and specialized structures, as in technologically advanced countries. *Culture* is the word used in sociology to refer to the way of life of a particular society, and cultural differences exist in even the most basic of everyday living activities.

Within the past few decades, however, a host of circumstances including emigration and the movement of refugees has accelerated a mixing of cultures so that within recognized national boundaries, multicultural societies are becoming more common. This introduces a fascinating diversity yet also holds the seeds of conflicting interests and potential unrest. Cultural idiosyncrasies related to a person's ALs are an essential dimension of the Roper-Logan-Tierney model of living.

Spirituality, religion and ethics. An aspect of living that is a reflection of culture, and which is sometimes overlooked, is spirituality. Murray & Zenter (1988) defined spirituality as: 'a quality that goes beyond religious affiliation; that strives for inspiration, reverence, awe, meaning and purpose, even in those who do not believe in God.' Labun (1988) defined it broadly as 'that which inspires in one the desire to transcend the realm of the material'. Discussing this definition, Labun (1988) maintains that it could refer to religion as well as more philosophical orientations to belief and meaning in life. The characteristics of the spiritual self, she goes on, in combination with those of the emotional and physical self respond to situations as a totality. As far as orientation to belief and meaning in life are concerned, these are reflected in ethical standards and manifest themselves in 'being true to oneself', as well as in behaviour to other people.

Organized religions can be considered as specific manifestations of spirituality, and are often closely linked to culture. In fact, for someone who feels alone and deprived of social networks that would give meaning to existence, religion can sometimes supply an identity, as well as communal links around religious observances.

A religion's influence on group and individual behaviour can be considerable; indeed, where there is religious unity in a society, the culture and religion are almost inseparable. Religion can influence ALs such as eating and drinking, eliminating, personal cleansing and dressing, and expressing sexuality. However, secular groups such as humanists facilitate their members' expression of spirituality in a number of ways which can affect an adherent's ALs just as forcibly as a recognized religion.

Community. As well as belonging to a society and sharing its culture, every person is a member of a community. The kind of community in which people live greatly affects the quality of their lives; even their personal safety is to a large extent dependent on the maintenance of safety in the community at large, for example in its schools and transport systems, at work, and in the provision made for the observance of law and order.

Role. The concept of role is helpful in describing the part an individual plays in society. There are many different social roles and each carries very specific expectations and makes specific demands on the individual. From birth, a male baby may occupy the roles of son, brother and grandson, and these differ from the daughter, sister and granddaughter roles of a female baby. These are examples of 'ascribed' roles, i.e. those allocated to people at birth according to their sex and existing kinship network. Others are 'achieved' as a result of personal choice and endeavour, for example occupational roles.

Status. Even such fundamental roles as man or woman and child or parent have to be learnt. One of the important functions of the family is the socialization of children, the process whereby they are taught and learn about the characteristics, expectations and responsibilities attached to the whole range of social roles. In general, there are differences in the degree of status attached to particular roles, and in the importance attributed to 'ascribed' as compared to 'achieved' roles.

Relationships. In any society, each individual has his or her own unique network of relationships. Initially, this emerges from the kinship network into which the person is born, and it comprises relationships with members of the nuclear family or step-family and the extended family, then in adulthood to relationships arising from marriage or partner arrangement, childbearing and an occupation. During adult life, a person's network continually changes and expands; in old age, there is a gradual retraction in the number and variety of social relationships. The concept of relationships is not static. In the past few decades, in most countries, social mores have changed and relationships that were once socially questioned have become tolerated and acceptable.

Social groups. However, an individual does not interact only with another individual. Cooperation plays an important role in a complex society and to this end a great deal of social interaction takes place within social groups. An individual begins life as a member of the most generic social group, the family, and the concept of family now has a wide interpretation. Thereafter, individuals spend their entire lives joining and leaving various groups which exist in society to serve a multitude of functions: social, occupational, recreational, educational, political, spiritual and religious. In general, membership of groups is extremely important for the fulfilment of love and belonging needs and the development and enhancement of self-esteem. Those individuals not strongly integrated with social groups may suffer from social isolation and become lonely and depressed, even sometimes suicidal.

Social stratification and social class. Almost every society, in addition to a set of social institutions, has some form of social stratification which delineates the role and status of its various groups. Social stratification results from a layering process which creates units described as social classes. A social class is a group of people who have in common certain social, economic and occupational characteristics which determine their relative social status within society. There are different systems of class used throughout the world. In industrialized countries, the class system is often based on occupational grouping, and in the UK the Registrar General's Social Class Scale has been used for many years to categorize social class according to occupation. Since the Second World War, however, there has been a marked breakdown in class barriers and, as a result of these changing patterns, social researchers are beginning to experiment with new ways of categorizing class. Nevertheless in general, people still tend to think of three social classes—'upper', 'middle' and 'working' class—and to attribute to each a stereotyped set of characteristics.

The concept of social class is useful in order to understand the variations in lifestyles of different social groups. For example, it is known that methods of child-rearing and the value placed on education vary between socioeconomic groupings. Power and status in society are also related to social class, those of the 'upper' socioeconomic groupings usually having greater political power and social influence. Whether or not there is the opportunity for social mobility later in life, the classification of a child is determined at birth according to the father's social position. In this and many other matters, it is the social institution of the family—even although nowadays in Western countries, the 'family' has come to have a much wider interpretation—that determines and shapes an individual's personal process of socialization, and therefore influences most of the ALs that interact to produce individuality in living.

However, although sociocultural factors have a considerable influence on ALs, individuals in a society are also influenced by the physical environment in which they live.

Environmental

The environmental factors differ from the other four factors featured in this model (biological, psychological, sociocultural and politicoeconomic) in that they do not fall neatly into the knowledge base associated with recognized disciplines such as biology, psychology, sociology and politics. 'The environment' is a much more nebulous concept; indeed, Albert Einstein gave a simple definition: 'everything which isn't me'! In this text, it is considered to include all that is physically external to the individual person, so the scope is virtually limitless and could include a multitude of circumstances, featuring in a wide variety of disciplines that affect the individual. Despite the potential vastness of the subject, however, there are some more obvious applications to everyday living and these are used as examples of the impact of environmental factors on living.

The atmosphere: light and sound waves. The atmosphere is all around us and has many properties that influence humans, some helpful and some adverse. For example, the atmosphere transmits *light rays*, most importantly from the sun. Of course, light rays can also be produced artificially by means of, for example, generators or batteries, making it possible to continue all sorts of activities in the home, for recreation, and for commerce and industry during non-daylight hours.

Light rays not only stimulate the sense of light in normal eyes, but also provide the ambience for various ALs such as communicating, so that hearing-impaired people maximize the visual input of a conversation; or for eating and drinking, when soft lighting can be relaxing; or for expressing spirituality in cathedrals and churches where candles may be lit to meet various spiritual objectives.

Of course, the sun's rays also provide the earth with energy and heat; some of them are absorbed by the earth and some are radiated back into space. However, gases in the atmosphere (carbon dioxide, methane, chlorofluorocarbons) may absorb some of this energy, forming a blanket which returns additional heat to the earth—the so-called greenhouse effect, about which there is considerable controversy. Adversely for humans, some of the sun's rays (ultraviolet) may burn exposed skin or, after long exposure, may even cause cancer, so many people require to take preventive action by applying screening lotion or wearing clothes that cover the skin—a relationship to the AL of personal cleansing and dressing.

Sound waves, too, are transmitted by the atmosphere and, in various ways, can influence different ALs. For example, those produced by speech are an essential part of communicating for most people. Sound may also be a means of giving information or providing entertainment via tapes, radio and television, or as a source of pleasure in the form of pop music, choirs or orchestral concerts. Sound, however, may become a hazard, for example excessive vehicular or air traffic, building construction noise or loud music. These are all a form of noise pollution which is not uncommon in modern living, and potentially cause deafness in varying degrees.

The atmosphere: organic and inorganic particles. There are countless particles of organic and inorganic matter in the atmosphere. Dust is everywhere and the minimization of dust is an important contribution to the prevention of infection in the home, as well as in clinics and hospitals. Organic matter in the form of pathogenic microorganisms can infect wounds or cause specific infectious diseases, and if fever is present will affect the AL of controlling body temperature.

Other pathogens cause inflammation, for instance in the intestinal tract as happens in food poisoning; they can settle directly from the atmosphere on to food or can be transferred to food by vectors such as flies, or by unclean hands. The three ALs most likely to be affected are eating and drinking, eliminating, and controlling body temperature. In the home, in the workplace, in a recreational setting and in healthcare facilities, there are many prophylactic measures taken daily—by the public as well as health professionals—to prevent infection and its spread, but one prime example is the importance of handwashing. This should be done to remove both resident and transient flora before handling food, after visiting the toilet and after handling excreta, for example a mother toileting a baby or small child.

Although the most obvious AL affected by atmospheric components is the AL of breathing, atmospheric components and characteristics can influence several ALs as illustrated in the following examples. The rarefied atmosphere at high altitudes, particularly the reduced oxygen content, does not only affect breathing: because it lowers metabolism, less energy is available for the ALs of mobilizing, and of working and playing. In addition, the environmental temperature and humidity may well relate to ALs such as controlling body temperature, sleeping, and working and playing. And, in a more dramatic way, atmospheric turbulence in the form of gale-force winds, violent thunder storms or hurricanes will certainly modify the ALs of maintaining a safe environment, and of working and playing.

The natural habitat. Any discussion of the environment inevitably involves comment about the local vegetation and related climate. Crops, trees and foliage may be an important economic facility or may be purely aesthetic but, irrespective of their purpose, they should be conducive to healthy living. They should not be contaminated by, for example, the use of toxic herbicides or the fumes and particles of matter produced by vehicular traffic when crops are adjacent to motorways. Indeed, contamination of crops and soil, in turn, may leach into rivers and oceans and affect the health of marine life.

But, apart from upsetting the natural ecosystem, any major contamination of the atmosphere, the soil and the sea by biological, chemical and nuclear pollutants can have an adverse effect on the daily lives of human beings by affecting a number of ALs such as breathing, eating and drinking, and maintaining a safe environment. The presence of an increasing number of pollutants in the environment is causing concern, worldwide, and there are many pressure groups as well as government agencies whose interest is 'to save the environment'.

Related to the problem of pollution is the fact that the world's commonly used energy resources—fossil fuels such as coal and oil—are dwindling, and internationally there is an attempt to conserve existing stocks. There is, therefore, a growing interest in the possibilities for commercially harnessing solar, wind and wave energy. In theory this would potentially reduce the amount of environmental pollution currently created by machines that use fossil fuels, and which continue to proliferate especially in the industrialized world.

The built environment. Inevitably buildings are an essential part of the environment and can influence several ALs. They need to be free from hazard so that their occupants can continue the AL of maintaining a safe environment. They should also be adequately ventilated so that inside atmospheric conditions do not unduly influence body temperature by causing it to rise or fall outwith the range of normal—an important factor at home, at school and at work.

In any consideration of buildings, of course, housing is of primary importance to the individual and can have a direct effect on the ALs. The availability of a safe, effective water supply and waste disposal system can affect the ALs of personal cleansing and dressing, and eliminating, not to mention the AL of eating and drinking; the adequacy of play areas inside and out-of-doors obviously is an advantage for the optimal physical and psychological development of children; high-rise blocks of flats with unreliable lifts can deter occupants from venturing outdoors if they are elderly or disabled, thus affecting the AL of mobilizing.

Solid objects in the home are part of the environment and they range from eating utensils to cooking apparatus, refrigerators, washing machines, television sets, furniture and furnishings. To ensure that such equipment is conducive to healthy living, including the prevention of accidents and, increasingly, the prevention of atmospheric pollution, many countries have evolved consumer councils or similar organizations to set minimum standards of quality and safety; indeed, many countries have legal requirements to regulate their manufacture and sale.

The condition of, and the facilities within, buildings associated, for example, with education, with employment and with recreation are, likewise, important. For all buildings, the aim is that, as well as being functional, effective, user-friendly and conducive to the health of users, they will also be aesthetically pleasing.

These are merely a few examples to illustrate the importance of the external environment when considering a healthy lifestyle, and when considering the individual's ability to engage in the various ALs. But, like the three factors already discussed, environmental factors cannot be considered in isolation: they are all linked to politicoeconomic factors.

Politicoeconomic

For the purposes of this model of living, the term politicoeconomic factors subsumes aspects of living that have a legal connection; frequently political and/or economic pressure and action is reflected in legislation. A few points are made here about their influence on some selected ALs.

The state, the law and the economy. In the modern world, every citizen is the subject of a state. The citizen is legally bound to obey the orders of the state and, to a large extent, the individual's ALs are influenced by its norms. These norms are the laws, and the state has the power to enforce the law on all who live within its frontiers.

The state is the apex of the modern social pyramid and has supremacy over other forms of social groupings, so, in general terms, the state regulates human activities of living. For example, in relation to the AL of mobilizing, traffic regulations are enforced by the state; and in relation to the AL of eating and drinking, there are laws controlling the type and amount of food additives permitted in food processing, and also regarding the cleanliness of premises where food is prepared which, in addition, involves the AL of maintaining a safe environment.

However, the state is dependent on the economic system that underlies the legal order; only limited social progress is possible when a state has a precarious economic base.

The influence of the state. The state has involvement, in varying degrees, with an enormous range of interests, some personal, for example the statutory requirement to register births, marriages and deaths, and others corporate, for example a legal structure to maintain law and order among its citizens, or the provision of national and local parklands for the leisure and enjoyment of all.

The power of the state is considerable. But if individuals are sufficiently outraged, they can register disapproval; examples of disapproval can be found in, for example, the suffragette movement, the pacifist movement, and opposition to the use of nuclear power, the contention being that when individuals suspect their rights are being threatened they will question the state. In many countries, these types of activities have contributed to a trend to decentralize some of the power of the state to a more regional level where decision-making can, ostensibly, take greater account of the rights and wishes of local citizens.

Certainly in a modern democratic society, individuals consider that, for example, they have rights associated with their ALs: the right to a safe environment; the right to work in order to earn a livelihood; the right to leisure; the right to health; the right to education; the right to freedom of speech, freedom of association and so on. But, while making such demands, citizens have to accept that rights and freedoms carry with them social responsibilities. They do not have licence to do what they like; they have freedom to act responsibly within the law and appreciate that other people have equal rights to carry out their various ALs.

The influence of the individual in the state. Of course the individual may not always be immediately conscious of personal political power vis-à-vis the state, but the combined efforts of individuals working as a group can have a profound effect. In the vast modern state, associations have come to assume considerable importance; indeed, some focus on their ability to translate the results of their efforts into legislation, for example employers' associations and trades unions. And many small voluntary groups, pioneering minority causes, may highlight issues that are precursors to legislation. Of course, all associations are not directly relevant to the state; they may be formed for the purposes of sport or for aesthetic pursuits, and add considerably to the variety and quality of daily life.

The welfare state. In varying degrees, the modern state is a welfare state, virtually ensuring for all citizens a minimum level of protection against social risks. The interpretation of 'minimum' is a political decision and is influenced by the country's economic status and level of affluence. Gradually, however, claims against the national budget have come to cover the entire lifespan, for example, for maternity grants at birth, for child allowances, for general education and higher education, during unemployment, for pensions at retirement, and finally for death grants. All groups in society have come to have considerable dependence on the state. However, in periods of economic recession, it becomes more immediately apparent that a national budget is finite, that competing claims have to be arranged in some order of priority, and that in the process certain demands, albeit worthy, will be unmet.

In fact, quite apart from periods of recession, many countries in the Western world are finding the welfare state concept insatiable in terms of cost. They are reappraising selected health and social services that have been free or offered at token cost and seeking to put some of the financial responsibility back to the individual and/or family.

The interdependence of states. In the modern world, the state is not concerned only with its own citizens. Each state is one among many, and some of the most important current issues are problems that are external to the individual state. It has come to be realized that it is necessary to have regulations between states in the form of international laws; rapid economic and political changes make it unsatisfactory to leave individual states to make decisions in isolation on matters that are really of international concern.

The world is now interdependent in a large array of matters related to, for example, frontiers, tariffs, marketing, labour laws, monetary markets, shipping channels and flight paths, as well as for health regulations; in varying degrees these affect each state and eventually the individual's ALs. Indeed, some of the politicoeconomic issues have ethical considerations such as the unequal distribution of food, a basic necessity for living; in many wealthy countries there is a superabundance, and in others the economic level of the state is so fragile that its citizens are undernourished and sometimes starving.

World interdependence, in fact, appears to be leading the United Nations Organization into a controversial sphere: the right to humanitarian intervention. This is a revolutionary concept in world affairs. It is not mentioned in the Charter of the UN; indeed, any sort of intervention 'direct or indirect, individual or collective' in the domestic jurisdiction of another state is explicitly banned. Yet the world seemed to applaud when, in the name of the UN, a 'benevolent' army of occupation entered Iraq following the Gulf War to protect the Kurds; went to Somalia in 1993; or was sent as a peace-keeping force to the former Yugoslavia—all attempts at maintaining a safe environment for the people involved or avoiding a spillover of violence to neighbouring countries.

In the post-Cold War world, calls on the UN increasingly result from the collapse of nation states, ethnic conflict, major humanitarian disasters or a combination of these. It is one thing to introduce a peace-keeping force between two consenting parties, but quite another to inject a peace-keeping force into civil war situations without invitation from the warring factions, and with little prospect of bringing pressure to bear on the opposing parties.

In fact, the UN lacks the money and trained personnel to enforce humanitarian operations everywhere they might be needed in the world, but the issue is creating international controversy and, sometimes, acrimony.

These few examples indicate that this vast interdependence, this globalization, has actually created a world community in political, economic and, to some extent, legal terms, operating alongside the national and local structures that have a more obvious influence on the individual's ALs.

In this section, the five factors (biological, psychological, socio-cultural, environmental and politicoeconomic) that can influence the ALs have been outlined. But, as indicated in Figure 2.1, all four concepts in the model of living contribute to the fifth concept, namely, individuality in living.

Individuality in living

Our model of living attempts to provide a simple conceptualization of the complex process of 'living'. However, the concern of the model is with living as it is experienced by each individual and this fifth and final component/concept, individuality in living, serves to emphasize this point.

The ALs were selected as the main concept of the model and, although every person carries out all of the ALs, each individual does so differently. In terms of our model, this individuality can be seen to be a product of the influence on the ALs of all the other concepts and the complex interaction among them. Each person's individuality in carrying out the ALs is, in part, determined by stage on the *lifespan* and degree of *dependence/independence*, and is further fashioned by the influence of various *biological, psychological, sociocultural, environmental and politicoeconomic factors*.

A person's individuality can manifest itself in many different ways, for example in:

- *how* a person carries out the AL
- *how often* the person carries out the AL
- *where* the person carries out the AL
- *when* the person carries out the AL
- *why* the person carries out the AL in a particular way
- what the person *knows* about the AL
- what the person *believes* about the AL
- the *attitude* the person has to the AL.

The idea that this concept of the model—individuality in living—is a product of the other concepts is conveyed in the way it is depicted in the diagram of the model of living (Fig. 2.1). The other four concepts combine to produce the unique mix that determines individuality.

Again, it must be emphasized that the diagram of a model is merely an aide-mémoire and, indeed, has little meaning without explanation. Although each of the five concepts was described separately, the fact that they are closely related was emphasized; the relationships are portrayed in the diagram both by position and the addition of arrows. In other words, the whole model is more than the simple sum of its parts.

Given our emphasis on the individual person as central to our model of living, ipso facto, a family—and nowadays this term has a wide interpretation—has to be viewed as a collection of individuals, so their individuality may also have to be considered. To aid thinking about and providing a milieu congenial to healthy living for a larger group of people such as 'a community', our proposed model of conceptualizing living is also a pertinent basis, because, as we have described them, the concepts are broad and can have wide application. The Roper-Logan-Tierney model of nursing is based on this model of living, and both were developed from a research project, as already mentioned.

REFERENCES

Fawcett J 1995 Conceptual models of nursing. Davis, Philadelphia
Kübler-Ross E 1969 On death and dying. Macmillan, New York
Labun E 1988 Spiritual care: an element in nursing care planning. Journal of Advanced Nursing 13(3):314–320
Murray R, Zenter J 1988 Nursing concepts for health promotion. Prentice-Hall, Hemel Hempstead, UK
Wiggens J, Wiggens B, Sanden J 1994 Social psychology, 5th edn. McGraw Hill, New York

3

The model of nursing

We believe that our conceptualization of nursing based on a Model of Living captures the 'core' of nursing (p. 9). It is an indisputable fact that people who are in need of the nursing part of the health service, for whatever reason and wherever they are located, have to go on 'living'; therefore our model of nursing is underpinned by the model of living. The rationale is that a similar mode of thinking engendered by the two models will encourage minimal disturbance of the pattern of living while a person requires nursing, unless, of course, the person needs help in learning to cope with a different lifestyle. Figure 3.1 illustrates the main concepts in both models. They differ only in the fifth concept. The objective in conceptualizing living according to the first four concepts in the model of living is to identify each person's individuality in living, and this is the basis of our conceptualization of nursing. The objective in conceptualizing nursing according to the first four concepts in the model of nursing is to identify the

MODEL OF LIVING	MODEL OF NURSING
12 Activities of Living (ALs) Lifespan Dependence/independence continuum Factors influencing the ALs Individuality in living	12 Activities of Living (ALs) Lifespan Dependence/independence continuum Factors influencing the ALs Individualizing nursing

Figure 3.1 Comparison of the main concepts in the model of living and the model of nursing.

individual's pattern of living (and actual or potential problems with any of the ALs) so that the nurse can individualize the nursing of that person taking account of that individual's lifestyle—and when appropriate, taking account of family and/or significant others. Individualizing nursing is accomplished by application to practice of the concept of the process of nursing comprising four phases as shown in Figure 3.2.

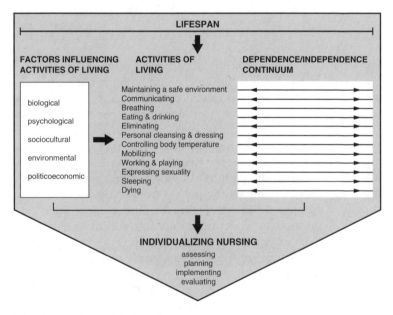

Figure 3.2 The model of nursing.

Our model of nursing is, we believe, sufficiently broad and flexible to be used as a framework for the process of nursing in any area of professional practice, whether in a community or hospital setting, and is a means of appreciating the underlying unity of the various branches of the profession. However, even more importantly, the person who comes into contact with the nursing service is central to the model, and the nursing required can be tailored to the individual's circumstances and not imposed by the nurses.

Certainly, the model *appears* simple—as simple as the model of living on which it is based. This is not to suggest that either 'living' or 'nursing' is a simple process because, of course, they are not. However, we believe that, to be useful, a model should be readily understood and, in the case of nursing, directly relevant and applicable to practice. There is no necessity for a model to exhaust every aspect of the subject and, indeed, if its presentation is excessively complicated by detail, its application to practice is unlikely to be readily apparent, however interesting and academically respectable it may be. Deliberately our model *seems* uncomplicated, but, as John Ruskin said, 'it is far more difficult to be simple than to be complicated'. Our model is offered as an overall framework to assist learners to develop a way of thinking about nursing in general terms, which then can be utilized in practice as a means of developing individualized nursing.

However, at this point it is appropriate to state the assumptions on which our model of nursing is based.

Assumptions on which the model is based

The selected concepts and their relationships in a nursing model are, as Fawcett (1995) said, a means of expressing 'the author's beliefs and values' which are a part of 'the philosophical foundations of a model'. We also believe that they are a means of interpreting the discipline of nursing. It is not surprising, therefore, that creators of models give considerable attention to the assumptions that underlie their approach to the discipline. The authors of the Roper-Logan-Tierney model make the following assumptions:

- Living can be described as an amalgam of Activities of Living (ALs).

- The way ALs are carried out by each person contributes to individuality in living.
- The individual is valued at all stages of the lifespan.
- Throughout the lifespan until adulthood, the majority of individuals tend to become increasingly independent in the ALs.
- While independence in the ALs is valued, dependence should not diminish the dignity of the individual.
- An individual's knowledge about, attitudes to, and behaviour related to the ALs are influenced by a variety of factors which can be categorized broadly as biological, psychological, sociocultural, environmental and politicoeconomic factors.
- The way in which an individual carries out the ALs can fluctuate within a range of normal for that person.
- When the individual is 'ill', there may be problems (actual or potential) with the ALs.
- During the lifespan, most individuals experience significant life events or untoward events which can affect the way they carry out ALs, and may lead to problems, actual or potential.
- The concept of potential problems incorporates the promotion and maintenance of health, and the prevention of disease; and identifies the role of the nurse as a health teacher, even in illness settings.
- Within a healthcare context, nurses and patients/clients enter into a professional relationship whereby, whenever possible, the patient/client continues to be an autonomous, decision-making individual.
- Nurses are part of a multiprofessional healthcare team who work in partnership for the benefit of the client/patient, and for the health of the community.
- The specific function of nursing is to assist the individual to prevent; alleviate or solve; or cope positively with, problems (actual or potential) related to the ALs.

It is evident that several of the assumptions apply equally to the model of living. This is not surprising because the input initiated by nurses is partly concerned with enabling patients/clients to continue attending personally to their relevant ALs; providing appropriate help, related to the ALs, when patients/clients are experiencing one or more problems; or indeed taking professional responsibility for the physical functioning of several ALs when a patient is, for example, unconscious. It is this flexible approach to living and to nursing which helps student nurses to appreciate that the Roper-Logan-Tierney conceptualization of nursing straddles boundaries which might be imposed by medical diagnoses, or the clinical label of the primary care facility, or the hospital ward or department specialty. And it goes without saying that, while concerned about a client's ALs, it is also important for nurses to consider their own 'living'—their own relevant ALs—while providing a nursing service.

Activities of Living (ALs)

As in the model of living, the ALs are considered as the main component of the model of nursing and they are illustrated in Figure 3.3.

The ALs (outlined on pp. 15–55) are the focus of the model because they are central to our view of nursing and characterize 'the person' who is central to the model. Nursing is viewed as helping people:

- to prevent identified potential problems with ALs from becoming actual problems
- to solve identified actual problems
- where possible, to alleviate those that cannot be solved
- to help the person cope positively with problems that cannot be solved or alleviated
- to prevent recurrence of a solved problem

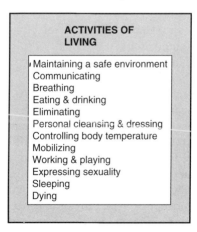

Figure 3.3 The Activities of Living.

- to help the person to be as comfortable and pain-free as possible, and maximize their quality of living, when death is inevitable.

Recognition of the fact that people's problems with ALs may be actual or potential means that nursing not only responds to existing problems but is also concerned with preventing problems, whenever possible.

The 12 ALs as described in the model of living (pp. 15–55) are the focus of the two models, so the descriptions are not repeated here but it is important, in the context of the model of nursing, to make some comments on the ALs collectively.

Use of the concept of ALs

Naming the general concept. In our early work in the late 1970s we searched for comprehensive and widely accepted descriptions of nursing. One of the well-known pioneers in this quest was Virginia Henderson (1969) who described 14 'components' of what she termed 'basic nursing care'—nursing activities. Roper (1976) in her research monograph used the term 'Activities of Daily Living' (ADLs), which at that time seemed appropriate, but it was also in the vocabulary of occupational therapists. After lengthy debate we selected and named 12 'activities', then realized that 'daily' was not applicable to all of them, so we coined the term 'Activities of Living' (ALs)—not nursing activities but the client's activities.

However, we cannot stress too strongly that our concept of each AL does not stand alone; it interacts with the other components of our model, and it is the interaction that results in individuality.

We deliberately chose to use the concept of ALs in preference to 'basic human needs', a concept that has been widely used in nursing, based on Maslow's analysis of human motivation. He identified several levels of human need: satisfaction of basic physiological needs provided motivation to rise through the levels of safety and security, love and belonging, then to self-esteem and to self-actualization. To some extent, this thinking is relevant to the concept of ALs but, unlike needs, ALs have an advantage for a nursing model in that many aspects of an AL are usually observable and can be explicitly described and, in some instances, objectively measured. It is not easy for the nurse to assess needs as such; it is less difficult (although still not easy) to describe a person's behaviour in relation to ALs.

Naming the ALs. The terms we chose to name the individual ALs also merit comment. Although anxious to avoid jargon, finding suitable names for some of the activities was difficult. The names of the 12 ALs were selected in an attempt to be consistent in emphasizing their active nature (therefore, 'eliminat*ing*' rather than 'eliminat*ion*') and their comprehensiveness (for example, although 'washing and dressing' is the more common term, we decided on 'personal cleansing and dressing' because it is all- embracing of the various activities subsumed within that AL). As a consequence, some of the names may seem rather strange at first but we believe that familiarity with the names of the 12 ALs should result in acceptability of our deliberately and carefully chosen terms.

The set of 12 ALs is unique to our model. Many of the activities are contained in other lists, but in addition our list contains some activities (such as 'expressing sexuality') that have not always been included alongside the more obvious activities (such as 'eating and drinking') despite the fact that they are integral to the process of living and, therefore, relevant in the context of nursing. In fact, in the first edition (1980) the inclusion of expressing sexuality was greeted by some with considerable surprise. Indeed, in the first edition even discussion of the AL of dying was unusual in the UK. How times have changed!

Complexity of the ALs.

The fact that each AL is highly complex because it subsumes a variety of activities was a point mentioned in discussion of the AL component of the model of living (p. 16). The point is worth reiterating here because it explains why, in the context of nursing, there is such diversity in people's problems and related nurse-initiated activities associated with each of the 12 ALs. This will become apparent from further discussion of nursing and the ALs.

Relatedness of the ALs.

The relatedness of the 12 ALs was also commented on (p. 16) and this too is an important consideration in the context of nursing. In the course of obtaining information (by assessment) about any one AL, the nurse is likely to find out a great deal about other closely related ALs. For example, discussion of eating and drinking habits can lead naturally to description of eliminating habits. A problem with one AL may well cause problems with one or more of the others: for example, mobilizing difficulties are likely to cause problems with other ALs, such as 'personal cleansing and dressing' and 'working and playing'.

On the other hand, when applying the model in practice, the identified problem of, for example, pain could be placed on a Nursing Plan in more than one AL. If the pain can be identified as being specific to the AL of eating and drinking, or eliminating, or mobilizing, it would be recorded with that specific AL. If it were generalized pain, we suggest it be recorded under the AL of communicating because pain is a subjective phenomenon experienced via the nervous system, which in our model is allocated as a biological factor to the AL of communicating.

To repeat, *a model should be flexible*; it is not a rigid straitjacket. It is intended merely as a tool that can be useful to the nurse in practice.

Priorities among the ALs.

In providing a list of ALs (Fig. 3.3), no attempt is made to infer priority. However, although every AL is important in the process of living, some are more vital than others. The AL of breathing must be considered as of prime importance because it is essential for all the other ALs and, indeed, for life itself. The notion of priorities among the ALs was briefly mentioned in discussion of the model of living (p. 55), and in the context of nursing is an extremely important consideration.

With the exception of the AL of breathing, there is no fixed order of priority among the ALs because, depending on the individual's choice and prevailing circumstances, priorities among the ALs alter. On the whole, however, activities that are vital to survival and safety take precedence over others in circumstances of acute mental and physical illness, and any condition that is considered to be life-threatening.

Relevance of the ALs

Closely associated with the idea of priority among ALs is the notion of relevance. Although the 12 ALs all have relevance to nursing, not all of them are necessarily relevant to all patients or to any one patient all of the time. For example, although it takes up much time in ordinary life, consideration of the AL of working and playing will not be relevant during a period of critical mental or physical illness. Or immediately after a myocardial infarction the AL of expressing sexuality will have a low priority, but quickly the person is usually concerned about general appearance, and before discharge from hospital may wish information about whether and when it will be safe to resume sexual relations again. However, for a woman having a mastectomy many aspects of that same AL may assume great importance, both before and after operation, and in the longer term too.

What is important is for nurses to be aware that different circumstances create different priorities and, therefore, to apply common sense and professional judgement (which comes from knowledge and experience) in making decisions about the relevance of recording information about each AL for every person. Any one, or indeed several, may not merit consideration at all during a particular episode when a client requires nursing intervention (for example, during a short hospital stay or day surgery); or may merit consideration only at certain points in a person's nursing plan.

ALs and the individual person

After this more generalized discussion of the ALs—all briefly described in the model of living (pp. 15–55)—it is pertinent to focus further discussion on the other components and concepts of the model and how they influence the individual's ALs, namely:

- stage on the lifespan
- level of dependence or independence and methods of coping positively with dependence
- factors that have influenced or are influencing individual lifestyle, categorized as:
  - ⌐ biological
  - — psychological
  - — sociocultural
  - — environmental
  - — politicoeconomic.

Again, it is worth repeating that, although discussed under separate headings, it is crucial to remember that these components do not stand alone; it is their interaction which determines individuality.

Lifespan

The reason for including lifespan as one component of the model of living has been explained previously (p. 55): each individual has a lifespan from birth to death, but its length is variable.

In a nursing context, the lifespan (Fig. 3.4) serves as a reminder that nursing is concerned with people of all ages: that an individual may require nursing at any stage of the lifespan, from birth to death. So relevant is the concept of the lifespan to nursing that some branches of the profession, and some professional qualifications, are linked specifically to certain stages of the lifespan. For example, midwives are concerned with the prenatal stage, birth and the immediate postnatal period; paediatric nurses and health visitors with the stages of infancy and childhood; and 'care of the elderly' is the current official category for 'nursing' elderly people.

Taking account of a patient's age—the fact that identifies the stage of the lifespan—has always been recognized as important in nursing. It influences all phases of the process of nursing (assessing, planning, implementing and evaluating) and is an important consideration in individualizing nursing.

The following brief comments on each of the main stages of the lifespan help to illustrate the relevance of this concept in the model of nursing.

Infancy

The first moments of life after birth are crucial and, here, midwives—or obstetricians or, in some countries, birth attendants—play a vital role. They ensure, for example, that the AL of breathing is satisfactorily established; that there is immediate opportunity for communication between mother and baby. Promptly the baby is dried and kept warm to prevent problems with the AL of controlling body temperature, and so essential to life is the AL of eating and drinking that the midwife may encourage the mother to suckle her baby at the breast very soon after the

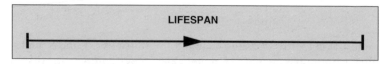

Figure 3.4 The lifespan.

birth although, for a variety of reasons, some babies need to have a breast-milk substitute. Helping the mother to learn to feed and care for her baby is a major concern of postnatal nursing, for after all the baby is totally dependent on the mother in respect of almost all the ALs.

Soon the young baby is experimenting with cooing and babbling noises, and eventually comes to realize that words have meaning. Talking to the infant, and cuddling and touching, which are all part of the AL of communicating, are forms of stimulation that are crucial to further psychological and social development; indeed, children deprived of these attentions over a period may have problems with future interpersonal relationships. Cuddling, rocking and touching are also pleasurable for the child and are an early form of expressing sexuality, although at this stage they are not viewed as explicitly sexual. Sleep is dominant in the early weeks and, not surprisingly, infants are said to have more stages 3 and 4 in the rhythm of sleep, when hormones are secreted.

However, throughout the first year of life, even the most healthy babies remain vulnerable to the hazards of infection and injury, and susceptible to a variety of problems with the ALs, for example hypothermia, malnutrition and dehydration. In all countries with a developed healthcare system, child health services are afforded a high priority and nursing makes an important contribution to efforts aimed at achieving ever lower rates of infant mortality and morbidity.

There are of course some babies and young children who, for a variety of reasons, require nursing in a neonatal unit or children's hospital. Their nursing is provided by specially qualified nurses who, in addition to knowing about the effect that disease can have on ALs, require an in-depth understanding of the normal processes of development in the early years of the lifespan. This is essential for nursing to be tailored to the very different needs and abilities of young children of different ages, and to prevent the experience of hospitalization from adversely affecting the child. There is now widespread acceptance of the need to avoid the adverse effects of separation, and for this reason parents are encouraged to visit freely and to take an active part in nursing their baby or young child.

Some young children have the misfortune to suffer from chronic illness or a fatal disease or a condition that results in long-term physical or learning disability. Frequent readmission to hospital and, in some cases, long-term hospitalization or community nursing support may be necessary. In such cases nurses play a very significant part in the child's early years of the lifespan.

Sometimes, babies and young infants die. This can occur at any stage for a variety of reasons. The desolation of parents requires skilful nursing and usually it is preferable for them to see and handle the infant before burial. It is salutary to remember that, in many developing countries, the infant mortality rate is alarmingly high, frequently as a result of infectious and diarrhoeal diseases.

Childhood

In the Western world, childhood tends to be a period of relatively good health for the majority, with death an unusual occurrence. The single most important cause of death in this age group is accidents: for toddlers, accidents in the home such as burns, falls and poisoning; and for school-age children, accidents when riding bicycles or engaged in sporting events. So, maintaining a safe environment in the home and during school activities is vital.

For children, play is a priority and is absent only in conditions of extreme deprivation. It is often spontaneous, but purposeful play is also important. Play can be exploratory, imitative, constructive, make-believe or involve games with rules. Play should be fun as well as a challenge, and toys are some of the tools of play.

Serious illness is rare. In childhood, apart from transient illness, such as respiratory infections or the infectious diseases of childhood, the majority of children have little need for medical treatment or nursing. The exceptions are those children with a chronic illness or long-term physical or learning disability. For nurses involved in their care, whether in the community or in hospital, one of the important considerations is to provide nursing in such a way that there is minimal interference with normal development in this stage of the lifespan, such as progress at school, involvement in family life and friendships, and increasing independence in all of the ALs.

However, even 'well' children come into contact with nursing through the school health service. Like health visitors with the younger age group, school nurses are primarily concerned with the monitoring of growth and development, and the early identification of problems, such as defects of hearing, sight and speech. The monitoring role of school nurses can include the daily activities of children with chronic bowel conditions, those with stomas, or with asthma. Above all, the role includes health education; children are introduced in a positive way to dental and oral hygiene; a well-balanced diet with controlled amounts of sugar, salt, saturated fats and fibre; prevention of infestation; sex education in the context of relationships and safe sex. In some instances school nurses provide treatment, but equally important is their referral of children and parents to an appropriate source of help.

Increasingly, health education is viewed as more than simply information giving, and through discussion, debate and experimentation children are being encouraged to appraise their personal health practices, to become familiar with the concept of preventing problems, and to develop positive health values at an early age. This is particularly the case in relation to drug and substance misuse, and also to smoking. Unfortunately even young children are subjected to peer group pressure to 'experiment', and health education efforts are not always successful.

A problem that is causing mounting concern in this age group is child abuse. Children, because of their vulnerability, are particular targets, sometimes from family members and friends, but currently also from paedophiles who may be part of an elaborate network of sexual abusers, and purveyors of pornography; information about contacts is readily dispersed on the Internet.

Adolescence

During this stage of the lifespan the dominant feature is puberty. Sex education in school and at home during the years of childhood helps to prepare the adolescent to anticipate and cope with the associated physical and emotional changes. However, for those who have been abused and 'kept the secret' (as often demanded by the perpetrator), increasing knowledge and experience during adolescence can give rise to severe feelings of guilt and lack of self-worth, and indeed the person may be scarred for life.

Many of the problems that can arise in adolescence are related to physical and psychological aspects of sexual development. Some adolescents experience severe emotional or psychological problems, such as depression or anxiety, which require psychiatric treatment; some require treatment for drug dependence; some may benefit from psychosexual counselling; some need treatment for sexually transmitted disease including AIDS/HIV. Many adolescents use family planning centres for advice about contraception and selection of contraceptives; and girls who do become pregnant may seek an abortion or require obstetric care. An unwanted pregnancy is not only a social problem; most young teenagers are ill-prepared for pregnancy, childbirth and parenthood. Thus it can be seen that a variety of nurses come into contact with adolescents: psychiatric nurses, nurse counsellors, school nurses, nurses who work in genitourinary clinics, and those in family planning services, gynaecology and midwifery.

For all of these nurses, an understanding of adolescence is essential. They are unlikely to deal effectively and sympathetically with an adolescent's problems, whatever they may be, in the absence of an appreciation of the emotional turbulence at this stage of the lifespan, and of other features, such as a teenager's changing relationship with parents, the desire for experimentation, the pressures of school and worries about future employment.

Appreciating these difficulties and remembering that adolescence is a period of transition, with fluctuation between the desire for adult independence and regression to child-like dependence, is certainly essential for nurses involved with adolescents who require home or hospital care, whether short or long term. Adolescence is, like childhood, a stage of the lifespan when serious illness is uncommon. For those affected that fact must make illness or incapacity harder to accept when it occurs, for example an adolescent who becomes physically disabled following an accident or an adolescent who is diagnosed as having diabetes mellitus.

Even short-term hospital care of an adolescent presents the nurses with a considerable challenge. On the one hand there may be the desire to be talked to and treated as an adult but, on the other hand, the circumstances may well precipitate some regression to child-like behaviour. This may be manifest in signs of fear and anxiety, or in a desire for parental closeness; or perhaps in a reluctance to accept responsibility and independent decision-making.

The swings of mood common in adolescence may make for difficulties in the nurse–patient relationship and ambivalent feelings towards authority may be projected on to nurses and doctors. Self-consciousness about physical development and relationships with members of the opposite (or same) sex may cause the adolescent person to experience considerable embarrassment in some physically intimate nursing activities, for example those related to the ALs of personal cleansing and dressing, and eliminating.

The death of an adolescent is uncommon and most are associated with sporting or road accidents, although in Western countries, the rise in the suicide rate for this age group is causing concern.

The nursing of adolescents, whatever the circumstances, requires sensitivity and knowledge of 'normal' developments in this stage of the lifespan. Whereas many health authorities provide specialist services for children and elderly people, very few such facilities exist for adolescents.

Adulthood

In discussion of development during the lifespan, adulthood is sometimes described as comprising three stages: young adulthood, the middle years and late adulthood. Here, all three stages are discussed together.

It is easy to appreciate the necessity of adapting nursing to the very specific needs and abilities of children of different ages. Adults of different ages also have special requirements, but because of their independence in the ALs and their relative ability to communicate their needs and desires there is not the same need to adapt nursing so specifically to age as there is with children and adolescents. It is also the case that the parameters of 'normal' are very much wider in adulthood, resulting in much greater diversity in lifestyle, abilities and attitudes than among children. Appreciating the diversity, however, is helpful because it warns against making assumptions, pointing to the need to collect relevant information about each adult person as an individual.

However, there are two dominant areas of concern for most adults, namely, work and family life (or other long-term relationships). Both are enhanced by good health and are directly affected by illness and hospitalization; therefore, individualized nursing must take account of the adult person's work and family circumstances. In some instances these circumstances may be directly related to the person's need for nursing: for example, someone who has suffered an accident at work; or someone requiring family planning advice; or someone requiring help with an emotional problem.

Therefore, work and family life not only bring adults into direct contact with nursing but can be directly affected, often disrupted, by illness and hospitalization.

Early adulthood, however, is considered to be a stage of relative stability, with both physical fitness and intellectual ability at their peak. Recreation (part of the AL of working and playing), whether a physical sport or a sedentary hobby, can be an important feature of young adulthood, bringing enjoyment and preventing boredom, and thus contributing to mental and physical health. Apart from those young adults who are continuing to cope with a life-long physical or learning disability, serious ill-health is uncommon and the death rate is low, although the AIDS epidemic currently affects this group most severely. Apart from AIDS, the more common conditions include bronchitis, peptic ulceration, gall-bladder disease, alcoholism, back injury and psychiatric illness, particularly depression. With advancing age into the middle years of life, ill-health becomes more common. There is a sharp increase in the death rate in late adulthood with three conditions responsible: heart disease, cancer and stroke.

Knowing the causes of morbidity and mortality in the various stages of adulthood gives some idea of the reasons why adults come into contact with the healthcare system, and with nurses. And this knowledge can be used by nurses, as well as other members of the health team, to encourage a healthy lifestyle, such as taking adequate exercise; eating a well-balanced diet and avoiding obesity; taking alcoholic drinks in moderation; avoiding driving after drinking; abstaining from cigarette smoking and eschewing drug/substance misuse. Health education is one means of encouraging adults to adopt a more healthy lifestyle and there are many ways in which nurses can contribute to this effort in both their professional and civic roles.

An important milestone in late adulthood is retirement from paid employment. Many people look forward to this event with pleasure as they consider the extra time they will have, for example to travel, to concentrate on hobbies or to seek new interests. For some, however, it is a negative event. It represents the loss of a meaningful lifestyle with its attendant role and status; the daily companionship of work colleagues no longer exists; and income may be considerably reduced. Many companies now have pre-retirement courses for staff in order to reduce the trauma and help people to fill the gap created by introducing them to a variety of potential activities to replace time spent at work, thus making the later years of the lifespan pleasurable and fulfilling.

Old age

Nowadays many more people are living longer. The World Health Organization (WHO) draws attention to the rising numbers of elderly people across Europe and the increasing proportion of the population over the age of 65 years, which is set to rise from 14% to 20% by the year 2025. In the UK, Age Concern estimates that at present there are approximately four people of working age (20–64 years) to each person over the age of 65 years, but it is forecast that in 40 years' time the proportion will be 2 : 1. These demographic changes are a matter for concern in terms of available health and social services. The incidence of illness in elderly people is known to be high compared with that in the rest of the population, so there will be greater demands on formal health services and the number of people needed to staff them; yet there will be fewer people, proportionately, in the 20–64 years age group to look after these increasing numbers of elderly people.

Despite the legitimately increasing concern, however, it should be kept in perspective because the majority of people in this last stage of the lifespan do manage to remain in their own homes, often totally independent (sometimes referred to as the *healthy elderly*). Much can be done, for example by the health visitor, to promote and maintain health in this group of citizens although there will, inevitably, be some in need of assistance with some of the ALs. For example, if living alone, they may have less interest in preparing a meal and may be malnourished; they may take less pleasure in grooming and, with reduced mobility, may take longer to dress and undress; they may lose interest in reading and in hobbies when sight and hearing are failing; thermoregulation may be more fragile, with a danger of hypothermia; their sleeping pattern may alter and cause concern.

The fact that ill-health is more common in this stage of the lifespan than in any other is reflected in the numbers of elderly patients in the wards of general hospitals. To some nurses this comes as something of a surprise and it certainly would seem to contradict the belief that old people are the concern only of the specialist services for care of the elderly. All nurses (with certain obvious exceptions such as paediatric nurses) nowadays require extensive knowledge of the process of ageing, a sympathetic understanding of the needs of older people, and a positive attitude towards their care and rehabilitation. Individualized nursing is as necessary for an older person as for a child or a young adult—even more so it might be argued, for there is a longer established individuality in living.

When physical or mental disability is such that an elderly person can no longer stay at home, or cope within a community care setting, placement in a 'continuing care unit' may be the only solution. In such a setting, the primary aim is to help the person to maintain what independence there still is in the ALs and, of course, to provide an atmosphere and environment that is like 'home' as far as is humanly possible. Long-stay care of the elderly has not enjoyed a good reputation on the whole and, while inadequate conditions may be to blame, staff attitudes probably contribute to the unnecessary routinization and institutionalization. Ageism, discrimination solely on the criterion of 'being old', has been investigated among nurses and others who provide a service in these areas. The emphasis nowadays on individualized nursing, through the process of nursing method (which is incorporated in our model) offers a way of enabling people in long-stay units to continue their individuality in living—their individuality in relation to relevant ALs.

The inevitable preoccupation of old people with death is something that should always be borne in mind by nurses who are involved with the elderly. It should be remembered that many of the older person's peer group will have died, and they often feel great desolation and isolation as they grieve for their friends and miss their companionship. In Western society most people die in old age, and skilled and sensitive nursing may help a person to come to the very end of the lifespan, to the event of death, in comfort and with the greatest possible dignity.

In this overview of the relationship between stages of the lifespan and nursing, various ALs have been mentioned, illustrating that the lifespan component of our model of nursing is closely related to the AL component, as it is to the dependence/independence continuum which will now be discussed.

Dependence/independence continuum

The reason for including the dependence/independence continuum in the model of living was described on page 57. The concept of dependence and independence has been widely utilized in nursing and, as a concept in our model of nursing, is related directly to each of the 12 ALs (Fig. 3.5). It is obvious that there is also a close link between this component of the model and the lifespan.

Childhood

Nursing for newborn babies acknowledges their total dependence in respect of almost every AL, whereas children's nursing must take account of the fact that the early years of the lifespan are associated with increasing independence in the ALs. Some children do not have the capacity to acquire this independence to the same extent or at the 'normal' rate, because of either a physical or a learning disability. Where nurses are involved in care of such children, whether at home or in an institutional setting, the objective is an individualized programme for the acquisition of maximum independence for each AL.

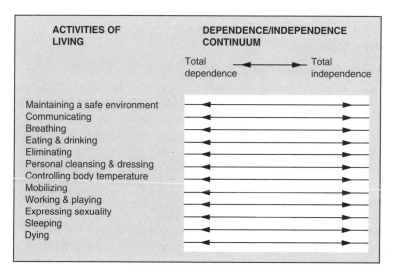

Figure 3.5   The dependence/independence continuum related to the Activities of Living.

For any child, an episode of illness or injury as a result of accident will not only affect the level of independence already achieved in the ALs but may also require a stay in hospital. Young children are very easily upset by any change in environment or alteration to their daily routine. For example, a child who has recently achieved independence in certain personal cleansing activities, or who is able to dress without help, is likely to be confused if the nurse washes or dresses them. On the other hand, children may be very distressed if expected by the nurses to exercise a degree of independence in the ALs that has not yet been acquired, for example being expected to use the toilet when still at the stage of using a potty, or being given a game to play or books to read that are beyond their level of comprehension.

It is obvious that nurses require to have detailed information about what each child can and cannot do independently in relation to each AL so that the nursing plan is tailored to the individual child, as well as to the circumstances of the illness or injury. As far as possible, children are nursed at home with support from the community team rather than being admitted to hospital. Or in some instances the child is discharged home and the hospital nurse visits, so that there is continuity of specialized care with minimal disruption to the child and family, and every effort is made to foster the independence of the child and the family.

Adulthood

For the majority of people, independence is a central feature of adulthood. When, for any reason, there is enforced dependence, for example as a result of illness or injury, many people find this hard to cope with. If the period of dependence in relation to any or all of the ALs is to be only temporary, for example following a surgical operation, it is likely to be more easily tolerated. However, if the circumstances mean that there will be some residual dependence in some of the ALs, the person needs time and support to adjust and to begin to cope with the changed dependence/independence status. This is particularly important when, for any reason, there is permanent paralysis and the person's mobility and sense of touch are impaired or even destroyed in certain areas of the body. It is also important when sight, hearing or speech defects impair the person's ability to communicate. Reduction in independence, especially when occurring suddenly, can drastically affect the person's masculinity–femininity status, causing frustration, loss of self-worth and a feeling of hopelessness.

Nowadays, particularly with pharmacological advances, people who have mental health problems may have only episodes of unwellness, and only during such an episode do they become less independent for some of the ALs. On the other hand, some require constant supervision by others to maintain their drug regimen—perhaps family members, perhaps community mental health staff—and, to that extent, they are dependent.

For people with learning disabilities, there are varying degrees of independence in the ALs, and support from family, health staff or voluntary organizations can help to provide them with optimum 'quality of life' standards.

However, when family members are the major carers, they too require support services from outside sources.

Of course, disabled adults are just as likely to suffer from the many conditions that bring the non-disabled into hospital or into contact with community services. So, when nursing adult patients who are physically disabled (or who have loss or impairment of sight, hearing or speech), nurses need to have detailed information about their dependence/independence status for each AL. It should not be automatically assumed that because people have, for example, a physical disability, they will necessarily be dependent on the nurse. They may well wish to continue to use the coping mechanisms, aids or equipment—'aided' independence—that have enabled them to remain independent in the ALs in their everyday lives, and nurses should ensure that this is made possible and that relevant information is provided on the nursing plan.

Old age

Even for the most able people, independence in the ALs is generally acquired over a long period of time. In old age the loss of independence can be equally gradual and it seldom occurs for all of the ALs. The AL of mobilizing is often one of the first affected and, because movement is required to perform many other activities, this may result in loss of independence in some of the other ALs. The elderly person may be reluctant to bath, and careful questioning may elicit that it is due to fear of falling. Difficulties with personal cleansing and dressing activities may in fact be due to problems with mobilizing. There are now many gadgets available to help elderly people with such difficulties, and provision of these may permit a person to retain independence, albeit 'aided' independence in these activities. It is worth repeating a point made in the context of the model of living that old age does not necessarily bring about loss of independence, and there is seldom dependence for all ALs.

As already mentioned, the age structure, especially in Western societies, is changing, and with a significant relative increase of those in their 80s and 90s, more provision is being made in the community for assisting elderly people to remain healthy and active, and to retain optimal independence. Clubs are available to encourage exercise, recreational games and handicrafts which, as well as encouraging physical and mental activity, also provide a social reason for meeting, and help to reduce the loneliness that often accompanies living alone. Especially in Western cultures with a nuclear family structure, more and more elderly people do live alone and currently there is a trend to provide what is termed 'sheltered housing', often purpose-built, where elderly individuals or couples, who are becoming less able physically, can retain their own home; however, each is connected via an intercom system to a warden's flat or telephone help service where someone is constantly on call. They are a form of 'sheltered independence'.

Discerning the level of independence

An important skill in nursing is developing professional judgement in relation to people's abilities and never depriving them, however old, of independence in those ALs for which they are capable. There is, of course, a fine line between this and misjudgement in demanding independence when a person is incapable of so being.

It is, equally, a skill in nursing to know when a person is in a state of dependence, or should be helped to accept that this is necessary. Although the emphasis in nursing is generally on encouraging people to achieve or regain maximum independence in the ALs, there are circumstances (for example, unconsciousness or severe mental or physical illness) when people are totally dependent on nurses. There are other circumstances when, although people may desire to be independent, this is not in their best interests. At certain times (e.g. immediately after operation), in certain illnesses (e.g. severe respiratory conditions) and for other reasons (e.g. immobilization in traction), it is important for the person to move as little as possible and for energy to be conserved. Such people may need to be helped to accept that their dependence is necessary and their distress is likely to be lessened if nurses carry out activities on their behalf in a willing manner and in a way that does not offend the person's concept of dignity and self-esteem.

Therefore, sometimes nurses help people towards independence in the ALs and, at other times, help them to accept dependence. The dependence/independence continuum in the model of nursing, as in the model of living, is arrowed to indicate that movement can take place along it in either direction—an important dimension of the concept of dependence and independence in the context of nursing. A very important aspect of nursing is assessing a person's level of independence in each relevant AL and judging in which direction, and by what amount, they should be assisted to move along the dependence/independence continuum; what nursing assistance they need to achieve the goals set; and how progress in relation to these goals will be evaluated.

There is little independent control over the *time* of death except perhaps in instances of suicide. However, nurses and carers can encourage the dying person to be as independent as possible whether at home or in hospital. It is important to recognize that family members or significant others may be transiently dependent on nursing skills as they work through the grieving process before and after the death has occurred.

Factors influencing the ALs

In the model of living (p. 59), this component was introduced to explain why there are many individual differences in the way the ALs are carried out. As described there, the various 'factors' that influence the ALs were categorized into five main groups, and in the model of nursing this concept is similarly presented (Fig. 3.6).

It is worth repeating that there are innumerable aspects of the five factors, and worth emphasizing that those selected for mention in this monograph are chosen because of their relevance to

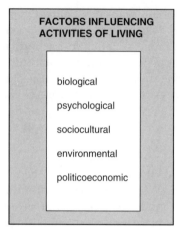

FACTORS INFLUENCING ACTIVITIES OF LIVING

biological

psychological

sociocultural

environmental

politicoeconomic

Figure 3.6 The factors influencing the Activities of Living.

nursing, or because they provide a context for the discussion of nursing.

As already indicated, the five factors influence each of the ALs and are related to the other components of the model: the lifespan and the dependence/independence continuum. The five factors themselves are interrelated, and, when assessing a patient/client it may be difficult to make a clearcut distinction between the influence of biological compared with psychological factors, or between sociocultural and politicoeconomic factors. Despite the overlap, however, the five factors are mentioned separately at this stage, highlighting some general points that are related to health and illness in a nursing context.

Biological

It is essential that nurses should have knowledge of biological factors and how they influence ALs. In the model of nursing, therefore, the status of the individual in anatomical and physiological terms is introduced to indicate how this helps nurses to understand, assess, plan and implement relevant nursing interventions and evaluate the effects.

There is no coverage of biological sciences in this monograph. However, to provide a context for discussion of the biological factors it is worth commenting on the nomenclature of various body systems and indicating how we relate them to our model.

Like all living creatures, the human body is made up of cells, about 10^{16} in number. In the human, although the cells are similar in structure, certain clusters of cells have become specialized to deal with specific activities, for example those dealing with gaseous exchange of oxygen and carbon dioxide in the lungs, and the cells secreting hydrochloric acid in the stomach to assist with the digestion of foods. Knowledge about these clusters of cells, or tissues, grew enormously during the twentieth century, partly because of increasing technical and technological sophistication in monitoring and measuring cellular activity.

At one stage in the development of such knowledge, the anatomists and physiologists categorized body tissues that seemed to interact structurally or functionally into body systems and labelled them separately, for example the skeletal, muscular, respiratory and circulatory systems. As knowledge developed, the interrelationship of these systems became even more obvious and terms came to be used such as musculoskeletal, genitourinary and cardiopulmonary systems. Thereafter, certain tissues with highly specialized functions were identified which previously had not been considered as systems, for example the immunological system, the temperature-controlling system, the reticuloendothelial system and the biorhythm system related to sleep control.

Obviously the human body is a highly complex organization of cells and tissues with many interrelated systems, so it is only for the purposes of learning and discussion that systems can be considered separately.

Given the complexity and the interrelationships, it is difficult to juxtapose just one body system with each AL; for example, although its main function is related to the AL of mobilizing, the musculoskeletal system is involved in many of the ALs.

One of the objectives in presenting our model of nursing is to help students to integrate, in this instance biological sciences, into the AL framework, particularly when the nursing documentation in use reflects our model. Therefore, to assist students to see the relationship of biological factors to ALs, we match a body system with an AL when relevant, for example the cardiopulmonary system with the AL of breathing; the lower alimentary and urinary systems with the AL of eliminating; the musculoskeletal system with the AL of mobilizing. It is not always possible to be so specific and three of the ALs are so generalized that they cannot be matched to a specific body system: maintaining a safe environment, working and playing, and dying.

The term 'biological factors', however, can cause a problem when mentioned in a nursing context. Some people still jump to the conclusion that it refers only to pathology. Unquestionably, nursing is associated partly with physical dysfunction and disease, particularly in emergency situations. But nursing is also concerned with the promotion and maintenance of health, and the prevention of disease, and it is imperative to have knowledge of the biological sciences in order to understand the normal structure and function of the *healthy* body.

Promoting and maintaining health. Irrespective of the setting—home, clinic, hospital—the nurse has innumerable opportunities for introducing aspects of health teaching that aim to maintain the body in a biologically healthy state. In fact, currently, in many industrialized societies, considerable amounts of money are used by governments via the mass media to extol physical health and fitness as a way of life, and the nurse as a health professional should not find it too difficult to reinforce the message. It should be borne in mind, however, that any discussion of promoting and maintaining health can provoke controversy; indeed, some people pose the question 'What right do health promoters have to intervene in the lives of other people?'. The nurse must gauge the appropriateness of introducing such topics—and know when to desist!

The biological state of the body is not static of course; it is constantly changing. Even during sleep the cells are perpetually active, and hormonal and chemical substances are regulating the body's internal environment to maintain homeostasis. It is not difficult to appreciate that for various biological functions there is a range of normal in terms of individual differences, and this is corroborated using physiological measurements, although even these vary with age, for example at rest a newborn baby has a pulse rate of 140 beats per minute and the normal rate for a young adult would be 70 beats per minute. It is within the range of normal that the body functions physically to its optimum.

Pregnancy is a time when most women (and some men) are willing to discuss the maintenance of health—for themselves and for the expected child(ren). For example, in relation to the mother's nutrition, a balanced diet is essential for the health of the mother and the growth of the fetus. Protein, calcium and vitamins are important constitutents and folic acid is currently known to prevent neural tube defects. Alcohol is discouraged; excessive alcohol consumption during pregnancy can lead to birth defects related to the condition known as 'fetal alcohol syndrome'. Pregnant women are advised to refrain from smoking: smoking is associated with reduced birthweight and also impaired physical and mental development in young children. Postnatally, the adverse effects of passive smoking on young children have been demonstrated.

Following pregnancy, the reproductive organs gradually return to their non-pregnant state and regular menstruation recommences within 3 months or so of delivery. But because the time of the first ovulation cannot be predicted, it is advised that contraception should be practised whenever sexual relations are resumed, as a further early pregnancy is undesirable. The availability of contraceptive techniques (mainly physical or chemical control of fertility) is considered by both men and women to be an important advance of modern times. Contraception allows women to exercise control over their lives and some would say promotes health by contributing considerably to their emotional and physical well-being. In some countries, where there is a problem of overpopulation, governments are active in promoting family planning (including the use of contraceptives) and educating people about the importance of birth control.

Promoting and maintaining health during the menopause is also important. For many women, the discontinuation of the monthly periods does not cause undue upset. For others, the decrease in the levels of sex hormones may cause symptoms such as hot flushes, headache, depression and fatigue, and sometimes loss of libido. Health advice and the treatment of such symptoms is important and make it possible to continue with daily living activities which are normal for that person. Although still subject to controversy, the therapeutic use of hormone replacement therapy (HRT) in maintaining health during and after the menopause is increasingly viewed positively. Apart from providing symptom relief, HRT has proven benefits in terms of reducing the risk of both osteoporosis and arterial disease in older women.

Preventing disease. Of course nurses are also involved in the process of preventing physical disease when, for example, explaining or participating in immunization programmes, and it is important for students to understand the physiological changes which occur in the body in the process of acquiring immunity so that people do not succumb to physical diseases which have the potential to cause dysfunction in one or more ALs.

Preventing problems and disease is also important in relation to the ALs of mobilizing and of working and playing; knowledge derived from the science of ergonomics can help to prevent muscle strain and pain when moving and handling loads at home, at work and at play. Quite apart from personal distress, back pain in particular costs industry millions of pounds per year in absenteeism when staff are on sick leave.

Another important feature of education about preventing disease is widely advertised in many countries. Smokers are cautioned about the known devastating effects, particularly on the respiratory and cardiovascular systems, when tobacco smoke is inhaled—and, as already mentioned, it may affect the unborn child causing fetal damage. The involvement of the cardiovascular system means that not only breathing is implicated: many ALs may be affected. Much effort is concentrated on the education of youngsters in order to prevent them starting the habit.

Drug and substance misuse is another problem that causes much concern in modern-day society, and the sequelae of prolonged drug dependence can be seen in many of the ALs. Peer pressure is strong and the excitement of risk-taking has powerful appeal especially to young people. The message of prevention has to be subtle to counter the seduction of the 'pleasures' these substances are purported to bring.

Physical disease. The desirable objective is to prevent disease, but some individuals may succumb to physical disease or trauma. This may necessitate nursing the person at home or in hospital during a brief episode of illness, or perhaps during the course of a long-term dysfunction or during the process of dying. Some of the causes of physical dysfunction are genetic in origin and some seem to start in a manner, not always understood, within the body's own internal environment, for example autoimmune and idiopathic diseases. As would be expected, when there is physical dysfunction in any tissue, for example caused by injury, infection, disease or irritants, the body does not remain passive; it reacts physiologically in a number of ways in an attempt to maintain equilibrium, via reactions collectively referred to as defence mechanisms. These mechanisms include the activation of the body's immune system; the protective inflammatory reaction following injury and infection; the process of tissue repair; indeed even the initial stages of the phenomenon of shock are protective, although obviously if not reversed fairly quickly such an extreme physiological reaction will have a fatal outcome.

It is particularly in relation to disease and medical diagnosis that nurses collaborate closely with medical staff; in fact, some nursing interventions, for example the administration of most medications, are still doctor-initiated.

Many diseases have been identified and rigorously researched and there is an internationally agreed Classification of Diseases which provides a yardstick, nationally and internationally, for the collection of epidemiological data about the incidence of disease and causes of death.

In all these instances—for the maintenance of health, prevention of disease, care during episodes of disease and during the process of dying—it is crucial for nurses to have a knowledge base of human biology and related sciences so that they can understand normal structure and function, and can comprehend pathological changes and the cause of dysfunction (in so far as it can be identified) and how it affects the individual's ALs.

However, as already indicated, ALs entail infinitely more than the body's biological structure and function; even basic survival would not be possible without intellectual and emotional abilities—the psychological factors.

Psychological

It is essential that nurses should have knowledge of psychological factors and how they influence ALs. In the model of nursing, therefore, psychological factors are introduced to indicate how this knowledge helps nurses to understand, assess, plan and implement nursing interventions, and evaluate the effects and outcomes. There is no attempt to cover the discipline of psychology in this monograph. General points only are made to show how this type of knowledge contributes to an understanding of human beings as manifest in their various ALs.

Intellectual development. Level of intellectual development, of course, influences learning ability, and communication (both verbal and non-verbal) is the basis of all activities associated with learning and teaching. To give a few examples, the AL of communicating is crucial in all child development and organized education; it will often determine employment opportunities; it is a powerful tool of the mass media; and it is a critical aspect of all health service interventions with the client or family.

To name another AL, a minimal level of intelligence is needed to acquire the manual skills of eating and drinking. It is also needed to select and prepare a diet to maintain health; the preparation involves knowledge of basic hygiene in handling and storing food, disposing of waste, and eliminating flies and vermin which can potentially contaminate food and drink.

In relation to impaired intellectual development, nurses may come in contact with children or adults who are mentally disabled because of a genetic disorder such as Down's syndrome. It is important, therefore, for nurses to know about genetics in order to be able to understand the principles of genetic counselling and the significance of diagnosis in utero via amniocentesis, ultrasonography or maternal blood sampling.

Knowledge is also required to ensure that a person with intellectual impairment is treated essentially as a healthy person, although pathologically slow in developing intellectual skills and the many other skills that are dependent on intellect. If a suitably stimulating environment is provided based on what such people *can* do rather than what they cannot do, it is usually possible to promote an optimum level of intellectual and emotional growth for each individual. Deprived of stimulation, the mentally disabled person may be grossly impaired and the effect on ALs is readily observable, for example in poor communication skills; difficulty with eating and drinking in a socially acceptable manner; problems with toileting; and incapacity for work and leisure activities.

Carefully staged education and stimulation of the intellect using an individualized plan is of major importance when someone has learning difficulties so that full use is made of the person's abilities, no matter how limited. There are many skills besides intellectual acumen that lead to a happy and fulfilling life. Reality must prevail, however, when discussing expectations with the parents of such children at the time of diagnosis.

Emotional development. Impaired emotional development is perhaps less easy to identify. The crucial mother–infant relationship was mentioned earlier: how it nurtures the growth of self-worth and how it influences the way in which the individual will eventually deal with emotions such as happiness, anger, fear, anxiety and stress, all of which can influence the AL of communicating. Each individual learns to adopt coping mechanisms, and for some people even apparently large amounts of stress are viewed as challenging, exciting and stimulating rather than predisposing to avoidance tactics.

On the other hand, in response to widely differing triggers, emotional reactions may be extreme and someone who is uncontrollably angry is more likely to cause non-accidental injury (NAI). This may be in the form of abuse to children, to women or to elderly people; or to rape and sexual assault; or gross violence to even innocent victims. The trigger may be excessive alcohol consumption or drug/substance misuse, although sometimes it is the result of a psychiatric disorder such as schizophrenia, especially if the person has defaulted on a prescribed drug. Several ALs are involved, especially the AL of maintaining a safe environment.

Psychological stressors are often associated with major life events and for some people may cause extreme anxiety. These significant life events may occur at various points on the lifespan; they may be developmental in nature such as weaning, toilet training, puberty or they may be associated with incidents in living such as changing school, job or house; marriage and divorce; childbearing; death of family members and friends. The anxiety may affect the performance of several ALs. In any of these situations the nurse may be asked for advice, and through counselling may help to prevent exacerbation of the cause, or assist the person to develop or maintain coping mechanisms until the cause of anxiety is removed or alleviated—and the person returns to a pattern of ALs that is acceptable to the individual.

It is sometimes said that psychological stressors involve the 'fight or flight' mechanism. For the purposes of survival, human beings are capable of an extreme response to perceived danger—an identifiable cause of fear. Activated by the autonomic nervous system and the secretion of certain hormones, there is an increase in heart rate and flow of blood to the muscles, a rise in blood pressure, and an increase in depth and rate of respiration. The body is physiologically prepared for fight or flight.

There are many life experiences that are less dramatic, however, and the physiological response is less intense, yet the person will describe a feeling of anxiety that may not have an identifiable cause. Because it is unpleasant, the individual may try consciously, or sometimes subconsciously, to avoid it. A range of coping mechanisms to reduce anxiety to a tolerable level can be manifest in observable behaviour and are important aspects of living; in psychological and psychiatric literature they are recognized as denial, fantasy, projection, rationalization, regression and withdrawal, to name but a few.

When, however, the stress is of great intensity and long duration, especially in a susceptible person who has not developed effective coping mechanisms, general systemic changes may occur and cause what are sometimes called psychosomatic disorders such as coronary heart disease, asthma and ulcerative colitis. Apart from adverse physical sequelae, some studies have shown that when an individual feels unable to alter the stressful circumstances, it leads to a feeling of hopelessness, and eventually pathological depression, categorized as a psychiatric disorder.

The effect on ALs can be far-reaching. For example, in a person who is pathologically depressed, there may be withdrawal from communicating unless pressed to respond; disinterest in eating and drinking; difficulty with eliminating such as constipation; disinclination for work or leisure activities; disruption of the sleeping rhythm, and so on depending on the severity of the depressed state. In some instances, there may be even attempted (or successful) suicide.

It is important, therefore, for nurses to have knowledge of psychological factors that influence ALs. It is important when dealing with a healthy person because even coming in contact with a nurse for advice on health, or for immunization to prevent illness, may induce anxiety. How much more so when the person comes into hospital. Not only is the individual anxious about the cause of admission: the strange environment also requires psychological adaptation to the disruption of normal patterns of living such as eating and drinking, eliminating, and sleeping.

The nurse must be sensitive to individual differences in the speed of adaptation to anxiety-producing circumstances. Slower adaptation is probably more evident at the extreme ends of the lifespan, and will require especially careful handling in our multiethnic society if the person belongs to a sociocultural group with which the nurse is less familiar.

Sociocultural

It is essential that nurses should have knowledge of sociocultural factors and how they influence ALs. In the model of nursing, therefore, social, cultural, spiritual, religious and ethical factors are introduced to indicate how this knowledge helps the nurse to understand, assess, plan and implement nursing interventions, and to evaluate the effects and outcomes. As already stated, there is no attempt to cover the various disciplines associated with the social sciences in this monograph. This area of knowledge is so vast and in any case, in recent years, there has been considerable mixing or blurring of social customs and beliefs among different cultural groups, partly because of modern travel, increasing emigration and immigration, and movement of refugees across national borders. So general points only are made in order to show how this type of knowledge (along with other subjects in the curriculum) contributes to an understanding of human beings as manifest in their various ALs.

Health status: effect on role. Different systems of health care throughout the world show that culture influences the way societies deal with health and illness. Deep-rooted cultural beliefs and traditions affect an individual's behaviour when ill; for example, responses to pain vary according to ethnic origin. Also cultural factors influence the way people treat others who are ill so that some types of disability and certain diseases carry a degree of stigma in some societies. Sociocultural factors are therefore important in understanding an individual's health behaviour and people's varied responses to illness and hospitalization.

Of particular interest to those involved in the delivery of health care is what happens to an individual's *role and status* when they become ill. Talcott Parsons, a sociologist, described this phenomenon as long ago as 1966 in what he termed the *'sick role'*. He pointed out that most societies exempt a sick person from some of their usual obligations and responsibilities as long as they fulfil a corresponding obligation to seek medical care and cooperate in the process of getting well. In many parts of the world there is in fact legislation to ensure that the sick are given special entitlements; for example, there are government schemes that provide the employee with sickness leave along with protection from financial hardship caused by loss of earnings.

However, as more recent writers have pointed out, there are many social implications of illness not considered in Parson's analysis. It does not acknowledge the subjectivity involved in defining 'health' and 'illness' or take account of the fact that some sick people will not get 'well' and others may not wish to co-operate in attempts to restore them to health.

Certainly, assuming the role of 'patient' involves many role changes; for example, a young mother is expected to receive rather than give care; the managing director usually responsible for many employees becomes the responsibility of others; and the lawyer and the labourer are treated as equals despite occupying quite different social positions in real life.

Health status: effect on relationships. It is not just roles that change during illness or hospitalization, but also *relationships*. For example, doctors' high social status is still reflected in the way some patients/clients tend to behave subserviently to them, submitting to their authority and accepting their advice unquestioningly. Such behaviour also serves to reinforce the traditional asymmetrical doctor–patient relationship. In fact, throughout the whole healthcare system there is an elaborate set of expectations and rules about the kinds of interaction considered to be appropriate between members of different healthcare professions and between professionals and patients, although this is changing rapidly.

In Western countries, many patients now want more than information: they want involvement in the decision-making regarding treatment options. Richards (1998) writes:

> . . . being confronted with a patient who has done a literature search, scanned the Internet, made a provisional diagnosis, and knows what he or she wants from the health service, is no longer a hypothetical scenario. People are becoming better informed about health, and a groundswell of support and government-backing exists for the campaign being waged by consumer lobbies, patient organisations and others for more and better information on health, and greater involvement in decision-making.

Inevitably in this context there are other patients/clients who do not have access to, or are disinclined to seek, information. So it is increasingly important for nurses to assess the individual's knowledge level of treatment options and their attitude to shared involvement.

On the other hand, there are still some developing countries where the extended family shares the responsibility and the physical task of caring for those in the group who are mentally or physically ill and/or disabled. This they do with few physical or financial resources, although there can be considerable emotional, social and spiritual support from the family, and sometimes the intervention of a local 'wise man/witch doctor' who may administer effective, though scientifically unproven, remedies.

Health status and social class. There is also an important correlation between social class and health status. In general, there are differences in the types of illnesses that affect members of different social classes. For example, statistics show that heart disease is more prevalent among professional people, and respiratory conditions are more common in less advantaged socioeconomic groups. Not only are there differences in morbidity, there are also differences in mortality rates: a baby born into a less advantaged home is more likely to have a lower birthweight and more likely to die in the first week of life, and there are strong links between social deprivation and premature adult mortality.

There is also an apparent correlation between social class and response to illness. The best possible use of health services tends to be made by members of upper socioeconomic groupings; others often fail to take advantage of provisions such as child health or family planning clinics. Sociologists have made a considerable contribution to, for example, the analysis of inequalities in health, thus assisting health professionals to understand certain aspects of the aetiology of illness and some determinants of health.

Health status and religion. The influence of religion on individual behaviour in relation to health and illness is a particularly fascinating aspect of the sociocultural factors, religious doctrines often dictating a very circumscribed lifestyle. Nurses are not expected to know about the intricacies of every religion but it is important to be aware that different practices exist so that every person's religious and spiritual needs may be appreciated.

Many religions have regulations affecting eating and drinking habits which will affect nursing activities. Orthodox Jews, for instance, consider every meal a religious rite and must eat specially prepared 'kosher' food at all times. Muslims consider the pig an unclean animal for food purposes and they observe total fasting throughout the daylight hours in the month of Ramadan. Of great importance to Hindus is cleanliness as bathing renders one not only physically but also spiritually clean; traditionally the right hand is used for clean tasks only, the mouth is rinsed out after each meal and the anal region is washed after defaecation.

Expressing sexuality is yet another activity of living sometimes influenced by religious beliefs and customs: limitations on family planning are imposed on Roman Catholics and Jews, and strict adherents of the Muslim religion prohibit free social mixing of the sexes.

A person's religious beliefs may also influence their attitudes to health and health care, and sometimes may present an obstacle to treatment. It is well known that Jehovah's Witnesses are not allowed to accept a blood transfusion and that Christian Scientists believe in the healing of illness by spiritual means. In fact, in the UK, religious and cultural differences may actually discourage the use of health services by people from ethnic minorities especially when there is also a language barrier.

For many people, however, religion provides a source of hope and comfort during illness. Sometimes, as in the Roman Catholic church, special sacraments may be offered to the sick and the dying. Baptism, thought by some to be necessary for a person's salvation, is carried out for any infant in danger of death or for a stillborn child (or fetus). The Sacrament of the Anointing of the Sick is often performed for a Roman Catholic during illness to aid healing and give moral strength or as a preparation for death. In general, for the dying and the bereaved, religion often assumes a role of great importance.

In fact religion, as a social institution, plays a key role in determining attitudes and customs on matters of life and death in nearly every society, regardless of whether the members actively practise the religion. In a multiracial society, some knowledge about a variety of religious faiths is a prerequisite for acceptance and tolerance of diversity in attitudes and behaviour.

Whatever the circumstances, the nurse offers care to people without regard to creed, race or skin colour. The nurse's function, generally speaking, is to provide an environment in which each person can continue to live by the principles that guide their behaviour.

Health status and spirituality. A concept that is more encompassing than organized religion is spirituality (see Model of living, p. 65). Interpreted as a 'search for meaning' in one's life, spirituality involves theistic and non-theistic approaches which can apply to agnostics and atheists as well as to followers of recognized religious persuasions. People who declare themselves agnostics or atheists may still require what could be termed spiritual care. During illness, a person with no defined religious belief may wish to explore feelings, values and life with another person, perhaps with the nurse as the person most available and most aware of the patient's thoughts and feelings.

Nurses need to consider carefully their own value judgements and accept that their personal belief system may not coincide with a client's system of beliefs and values. It is important to acknowledge that, for those who do not believe in an afterlife, death is an endpoint, and secular forms of funeral services may be desired by those who profess atheism or agnosticism.

It is interesting that the effect of religion and spirituality on mental health has prompted the American Psychiatric Association (APA) to include religious and spiritual problems in the *Diagnostic and Statistical Manual of Mental Disorders* (DSM-IV) under a broad section 'Other conditions that may be a focus of attention'. The Manual considers it can be used:

. . . when the focus of clinical attention is a religious or spiritual problem. Examples include distressing experiences that involve loss or questionning of faith; problems associated with conversion to a new faith; or questions of other spiritual values which may not necessarily be related to an organized church or religious institution . . .

The Deputy Medical Director of the APA enlarged that there is a need to be more systematic and inclusive with the category of conditions not considered mental disorders but which might be a reason for a person to consult with a mental health professional (Charatan 1994).

Health status: ethical aspects. Inevitably, as it is dealing with human beings, health care has ethical aspects. Since the compilation of the Hippocratic Oath in 420 BC, doctors have attempted to arrive at common principles of ethics in health care, but nurses and other health professional groups have also sought common principles to guide their practice, for example the International Council for Nurses has devised a Code for Nurses. In essence, such codes concern themselves with, for example, duty to do good and no harm; respect for life and human dignity; justice to individuals such as non-discrimination on the basis of race, sex, religion, political affiliation, social standing, disability and mental disorder; equal opportunity in terms of access to resources including preventive and treatment services; duty to protect the vulnerable.

The acceptance of such principles and putting them into practice will depend on the nurse's culture and type of experience, and the kinds of criteria used for interpreting, applying and justifying them. One instance of such a dilemma relates to the controversy over emergency resuscitation. Should this technique be used in every instance when breathing and heart rate appear to have ceased? Or are there some instances when the individual should be allowed to die with dignity instead of attempting to prolong an existence where there is no longer any quality of life? There are issues related to this particular ethical dilemma such as 'living wills' (advance directives) and euthanasia, and they continue to engender considerable controversy. They are mentioned in the Model of living (p. 51).

In this section, some of the concepts associated with sociocultural aspects of nursing have been mentioned in order to provide a framework for understanding some of the differences in behaviour found in individuals who require nursing intervention.

Environmental

As in the model of living, environmental factors cannot be considered in isolation in the model of nursing. They are necessarily related to the other components of the model of nursing; for instance a person's stage on the lifespan will influence the type of relevant environmental information required when assessing, planning, implementing and individualizing a nursing plan. The same applies regarding a person's status on the dependence/independence continuum. Knowledge from other parts of the curriculum needs to be synthesized into a nursing context so that, when possible, the environment can be manipulated to achieve people's optimal level of independence for carrying out their ALs.

The atmosphere: light and sound waves. In the model of living, the presence of *light* rays in the atmosphere was mentioned; usually light is considered to be a desirable feature. Nevertheless nurses should remember that what may seem normal lighting can, for some people, be excessive and distressing. It can be tiring for people who are ill, and prevent them from resting and relaxing or even sleeping; and it can be particularly disturbing for people who have photophobia or who are dying.

However, light has many positive uses in a health context, for example to assist in the examination of body orifices. Light from an auroscope is used to examine the external auditory canal which can reveal conditions interfering with hearing, and thereby communicating. Similarly, an ophthalmoscope is used to examine the eye, with the objective of identifying conditions that interfere with sight, which is also associated with communicating. Yet another example is the bronchoscope for investigating the bronchi when a person is experiencing problems related to breathing.

In more recent years, light transmitted through flexible glass fibres (fibreoptics) has permitted the use of 'minimal access' or 'minimally invasive' surgery (keyhole surgery), as well as extending the scope of diagnostic techniques. 'Keyhole' procedures are much less invasive, can sometimes be performed on a day basis, and may require only a local anaesthetic so are potentially less distressing to the patient and less disruptive to daily living.

Sound waves as a component of atmosphere need special consideration in a nursing context. It scarcely requires research to show that noise in hospital wards interferes with sleeping and ipso facto with resting and relaxing. But noise can also be intrusive and interfere with communicating when, for example, a nurse and a patient are discussing sensitive information. And it can lessen the concentration (a dimension of communicating) necessary when a disabled person is relearning mobilizing skills, for example.

Of course, noise can mean different things to different people. Indeed, it is possible to be upset by silence, for example a child in an isolation unit—a salutary reminder of the importance of individualizing nursing according to the circumstances.

The atmosphere: organic and inorganic particles. As far as organic and inorganic particles in the atmosphere are concerned, the whole philosophy and relevant action related to the prevention and treatment of infection can be applied to the model of nursing. This was mentioned in the model of living (p. 69), and prophylactic measures taken in the home, in the workplace and in recreational settings can be reinforced when the nurse is making home visits or when engaged in health teaching activities in the clinic and in the hospital.

As far as hospitals are concerned, almost inevitably there is a concentration of pathogens in such buildings and particular care must be taken to prevent their spread in circumstances where the debilitated immune systems of ill patients make them more susceptible; there is considerable concern about the incidence of hospital-acquired infection (HAI) especially when the responsible pathogens are known to be drug resistant.

The particle content of the atmosphere in the workplace also requires monitoring. When the work environment involves exposure to industrial waste particles such as the inhalation of minute asbestos particles or coal dust, or the handling of chemical or nuclear substances, special precautions are needed. In the UK, for example, there are now detailed codes of practice to protect employees from such hazards, and industrial health personnel, including nurses, have a responsibility for their implementation, partly through health education of staff. At international level, the International Labour Organization (ILO) has taken measures to encourage governments to provide employees with protection, including specially designed clothing.

The natural habitat. In the model of living, vegetation and climate were mentioned as examples of natural resources in the environment that influenced human lifestyle. In relation to the model of nursing, the use of crops and local foliage as a food source has relevance in varying degrees to human existence (depending on the family's economic status and/or the state of the national economy) and obviously is related to the AL of eating and drinking. In fact, almost two-thirds of the world's population depend on local produce, so the geographical position, soil, climate and rainfall affect productivity. In a fragile economy, failure of a crop, for example because of excessive flooding or drought, may mean malnutrition or even starvation. Not only is there food loss, but drinking water supplies may dwindle during drought and even basic sewage disposal systems may be destroyed during flooding, so that diarrhoeal epidemics are a potential sequel for the community affected. Especially in developing countries, community nurses are among the front-line workers who cope with the health aspects of such catastrophes by taking measures to prevent the spread of infection, tending to those who succumb to these adversities, and helping with food and water distribution during the emergency.

As far as environmental temperatures are concerned, and despite the human body's remarkable capacity to adjust to atmospheric changes, control of body temperature may become a problem. In very high environmental temperatures, children are particularly susceptible to hyperthermia, and in cold climates the problem at both ends of the age scale may be hypothermia.

The built environment. The buildings that are relevant in a nursing context are the person's home, nursing homes, clinics, health centres and hospitals. People's homes are relevant on two scores: firstly, should a member of the family require nursing services at home because of illness, the suitability of the physical layout of the rooms in relation to the problematic ALs needs consideration, as well as the availability of lay helpers, usually family members. If the person is very breathless or very ill and the house is on two floors, it may be advisable to put the bed in a room that is on the same floor as the toilet/bathroom. Discussion with the family will help them to make appropriate decisions about how ALs such as personal cleansing and dressing, and eliminating, will be carried out.

Secondly, if ill in hospital, it is appropriate to discuss with patients, before discharge, relevant details about the physical layout of their home related to the affected ALs, for example the availability of the toilet if the person has been prescribed diuretics.

Environmental facilities available at clinics and health centres can certainly influence several ALs. Clients with an increased frequency of micturition will need to have easily accessible toilets, clearly labelled. Inaccessibility for people with mobilizing problems may deter them from seeking help—it may be with a variety of ALs. Inadequate provision for pushchairs, cycles and cars can deter a wide range of people from seeking help because of inadequate transport and access, for example parents with young children, as well as disabled drivers of cars.

Environmental facilities inside hospitals and nursing homes are also important. The items of furniture, furnishings and pieces of equipment of necessity must be functional and designed for safe use but they should also be aesthetically pleasing. A consideration of bedclothes is important. More obviously they can influence the AL of controlling body temperature but they may also be associated with the AL of maintaining a safe environment: pathogens adhere to the scales of the skin's outer layer and are continually being shed on to the sheets. When disseminated into the atmosphere during bedmaking, they can be a cause of HAI.

Another important environmental feature inside the hospital and nursing home is the presence of plants and flowers. When brought by visitors, they communicate to the patient emotions such as love, affection, belongingness, being valued as a person and so on. They are also aesthetically pleasing and may evoke a response which, for some people, borders on spirituality.

Hospitals, just like other buildings, reflect the period in which they were constructed. When older hospitals were built, many patients remained in bed for most of the day, so their bathing and toilet facilities are inadequate to cater effectively for the needs of today's mobile patients. The same applies to storage space for clothes. For medium and long-stay patients, it is important to be able to store several sets of daytime clothes in order to allow for decision-making regarding general appearance, an aspect of the AL of expressing sexuality. Matching clothes to mood also helps to prevent conditions such as boredom and institutionalization. In older hospitals, too, adequate and pleasant surroundings for ambulant patients' leisure activities, and for eating and drinking, are often at a premium; these environmental factors can influence, for example, the ALs of communicating, eating and drinking, and working and playing.

The need for finance to upgrade older hospitals or pay for new buildings and equipment that provide a suitable environment for attending to ALs is one example of the link between environmental and politicoeconomic factors, presented in the following section.

In discussing environmental aspects of the ALs, scores of instances could be cited to show how they affect the various ALs. A few examples have been given to illustrate the relevance to the ALs of breathing, eating and drinking, eliminating, controlling body temperature, and mobilizing. However, users of the Roper-Logan-Tierney model of nursing will recognize other applications that are appropriate to their particular circumstances.

Politicoeconomic

It is essential that the nurse should have some knowledge of politicoeconomic (including legal) factors and how they influence ALs. In the model of nursing, therefore, political, economic and legal factors are introduced to indicate how this helps nurses to understand, assess, plan and implement nursing interventions, and evaluate the outcomes. There is no attempt to cover these disciplines in this monograph. General points only are made to show

how this type of knowledge (along with other subjects in the nursing curriculum) contributes to an understanding of human beings as manifest in their various activities of living.

Health and economic status. Conventionally, health has been considered to be the primary responsibility of the health professions and they are credited with improvements in health and the fight against disease. They deserve some of the accolade. It is increasingly recognized, however, that the major determinants of health are firmly rooted in prevailing political, economic and social realities; that health is not only a concern of the health service but an issue related to all fields of public policy. For example, the economic status of the mass of the population in a country undoubtedly affects living conditions and ALs, which in turn influence health and the incidence of illness.

It is difficult to appreciate just how precarious life could be for the masses in the Western world around 100 years ago. For example, at the end of the nineteenth century, life expectancy (one indicator of health status) for a male child in the UK at birth was 41 years, and for the female was 45 years (it is now 74 and 79 years respectively). As the result of continuing industrialization, the population was still adapting to the new urban way of life and experiencing new economic problems created by the growth of industry and decline in agriculture. The hastily built towns with poor planning, overcrowding, unsafe water supplies (AL of eating and drinking) and inadequate sanitation (AL of eliminating) were not conducive to the maintenance of health, and the long hours of work (AL of working) for low wages in poorly ventilated factories and mines, with unguarded machinery, accounted for crippling disabilities due to accidents (AL of maintaining a safe environment) and a lowered resistance to many of the prevalent infections. However, this began to change.

Health and political/legal activity. In the late nineteenth century there was an enormous sanitary reform movement which, with political support, culminated in the UK in the 1875 Public Health Act. The UK was not alone in the field of health reform. Around this time most other industrialized countries were taking similar legal action; indeed there was beginning to be international co-operation in an attempt to control the various pandemics— national boundaries were no barrier to the spread of infection.

Around the same period, too, in a number of industrialized countries, there was considerable political activity, which, along with the wealth that accompanied the economic industrial boom was focused to improve housing, to provide safer food, and to create facilities for better education. As a result of these better living conditions there was a decline in the incidence of several killer infections and the health status of the masses began to improve even before the discovery of specific preventive and curative measures in the form of immunization and pharmaceutical products. In factories, working conditions were also improved.

Health in industrialized countries. Much of the industrialized world's economic success which was reflected in environmental reform and improved health was associated with acts of parliament. National parliamentary action, however, was sometimes precipitated by the work of voluntary organizations, often working at a local level, not on a nationwide basis. Voluntary organizations did a considerable amount to improve health and well-being, for example by providing free milk for children (the AL of eating and drinking) or warm clothes (the AL of personal cleansing and dressing), or free contraceptives (the AL of expressing sexuality) to mothers who did not have the finance to support yet more children. When responsibility for making basic provision for such activities of everyday living was taken over by the government, it was possible to contribute to the promotion of health on a national scale. It is fascinating to compare the current position in the so-called developing countries.

Health in developing countries. When the United Nations Organization was established in 1945, many of the developing countries had the same major objectives as the industrialized countries cherished a century before: to develop the economic and social status of their peoples. The major emphasis was on economic development and investment in modern science and technology. An important economic asset in any country, of course, is the health of the workforce, but during the 1970s, the World Health Organization (WHO)—the health agency of the United Nations Organization—was showing increasing concern about the lack of improvement in the health status of the world's poorer, mainly rural, population. It began to be accepted that not only the conventional health professionals were involved in health: an integrated approach was required at government level from, for example, housing, public works, agriculture and education. Even more significantly, the community-based preventive and health promotive services needed the active participation of the people; to achieve this, political will and cooperation were needed at national and local levels.

Health and the world economy. Of course it is a rare nation that is economically self-sufficient nowadays. Countries and governments are economically interdependent and inexorably intertwined politically. The economic interdependence of richer and poorer nations was graphically described in 'North-South; a programme for survival'—the Brandt Report, produced in 1980—and it is tempting to think that in the intervening years progress has been made in some areas as irresistible globalization has proceeded apace.

The ending of the 'Cold War', which dominated international affairs for four decades during the twentieth century, certainly gave opportunities for a widespread discussion about democracy and development. In Europe, however, the threat of war was replaced by the threat of an uncertain future including hostilities between ethnic and religious groups; internationally, an economic recession made it difficult for developing countries to benefit from a potentially more peaceful world where, theoretically, less money would be allocated to military expenditure and more spent on health and economic development.

Inevitably, health and development are also linked with population trends and the estimated poverty level. Recent studies by the World Bank, the United Nations and the Organization for Economic Cooperation and Development (OECD) indicate that the number of people living below poverty level has increased because of the rapid growth in population. The 1999 Report of the United Nations Population Fund indicates that, since 1960, the world's population has doubled, and in Africa has trebled. Each year, the global population swells by 78 million—about 213 700 per day. Other studies in Europe and North America have found that the elderly, typically, account for 30–40% of bed-days in hospitals and of visits to family doctors, quite disproportionate to their percentage of the population.

However, even if population trends were ideal, the fragile world economy would not be helped by the fact that the developed world is moving out of an industrial economy to a biotechnological economy where robots are already doing the routine, manual chores at the workplace and even in the home—and sophisticated computers accelerate enormously the speed with which information can be retrieved and disseminated. The need for human intervention as a workforce contributing to the economy has been considerably reduced.

Politicoeconomic influences affecting the individual's health. Clearly the economic and social circumstances of an individual's community and the political will of the state exert a considerable influence on the lifestyle and health status of the individual and the family unit, and this will vary from country to country. As an example, in the UK, in the formal health service as such, political and economic circumstances influence the legal provision, and parliamentary acts enforce the registration of qualified practitioners such as nurses and doctors.

Parliamentary acts and legal requirements not only influence the practitioners in the health service: patients are also involved. Patients with certain types of disorders are protected by the law, for example in the UK, Mental Health Acts focus on the rights of mentally ill people especially regarding consent to treatment.

In the UK, too, as well as having government regulations related to the practice of the professional groups employed, and to certain groups of patients, the health service itself is still a nationalized institution, funded by government and influenced by the economics of the national budget. Of necessity, the financial allocation to health is finite, yet with technological advances making cure possible for increasingly esoteric disorders, the demand for the relevant expensive treatment is prodigious and cannot always be met, thereby creating considerable ethical dilemmas for both professionals and politicians. Most industrialized countries have similar regulations for similarly organized health services, and for the professional staff who work in them.

So, to understand the patient's circumstances and the nurse's legal duties and responsibilities, the nurse must have background knowledge of the political and economic factors that can, potentially, influence the individual's ALs, and also influence the nurse's professional interventions in helping individuals to practise their ALs in a manner acceptable to the individual and the community.

Individualizing nursing

The process of nursing. Individualizing nursing is accomplished by using the process of nursing which involves four

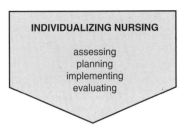

Figure 3.7   Individualizing nursing.

phases: assessing, planning, implementing and evaluating (Fig. 3.7). 'The process' is neither a 'model' nor a 'philosophy', as it is sometimes described, but simply a method of logical thinking and it needs to be used with an explicit nursing model. This is the rationale for incorporating the process into our model of nursing.

We have already stated the rationale for using the model of living as a basis for our model of nursing, and the patient's individuality in living should be borne in mind in all four phases of the process.

Patient participation in the process of nursing. Throughout the process the patient should, wherever possible, be an active participant, for example making decisions about continuing to carry out certain ALs and perhaps agreeing to modify others in the interests of health and recovery from illness. Encouraging a sense of personal responsibility for health, and protecting autonomy even in illness, are increasingly seen as important principles in modern health care, hence the emphasis on viewing the person as a 'consumer'—or user—and an active participant. Of course, participation may not be possible in the case, for example, of a child, a confused or an unconscious person. In these instances family members or significant others may participate in decision-making on behalf of the patient, possibly carrying out some of the ALs, as is usually the case when people are nursed in their own homes.

Patient participation demands a somewhat radical approach to nursing by both patients and nurses. To take patients first: in the past the majority accepted what happened to them while they were in the healthcare system, assuming that the doctors and nurses 'knew best'. With the social changes that have occurred in the past few decades, particularly the influence of the mass media, more and more patients are knowledgeable about what is happening to them and wish to be involved in discussions and decisions about their health and treatment. However, there are still people who are not sufficiently assertive to indicate their desire to be so involved and others who do not wish to be so, and these variations need to be recognized and acted on accordingly by the nurse, whether in relation to mental illness or physical illness. It is important to be especially perceptive when speaking with people who have learning or language difficulties.

Patient participation has repercussions in nursing which also require recognition. For example, the introduction of a policy allowing self-medication has obvious advantages for patients in terms of independence and preparation for discharge home; but, at the same time, this policy alters the nurse's role to one of teacher and supervisor rather than the traditional administrator of drugs. Understandably, careful planning and cooperative teamwork, particularly with the pharmacist, are essential.

The interactive nature of the process of nursing. Having made some general comments about the process of nursing, some more specific commentary is provided on each of the four phases involved. Although the process is described as comprising four phases, this is merely for the purpose of description and discussion. The implication in describing four phases is that they are carried out sequentially but in reality *all four phases are interactive*. It is important for nurses to realize this from the outset so that thinking will not be rigid and compartmentalized because, in practice, the process operates dynamically and interactively with *continuous feedback*.

Assessing

The word 'assessment' has generally been adopted for the first phase of the process of nursing. However, we think that overuse of the word assessment encourages the idea that it is a once-only activity and we prefer to use 'assessing' to encourage recognition of the ongoing nature of the activity. There is some dubiety about what assessing includes, so to clarify our use of the word, it includes:

- collecting information from or about the person
- reviewing the collected information
- identifying the person's problems with ALs
- identifying priorities among problems.

The information will be gained by observing, interviewing, examining, measuring and testing as appropriate; data gained at the initial assessment form a baseline against which further information can be compared. It is likely that, as rapport with the person is established, more information will be volunteered and, indeed, new and supplementary information becomes available to the nurse in the course of each contact with the person.

The primary source of information about the person is the person. However, secondary sources such as health records and family members are important and especially so in the case of children and disoriented, unconscious or severely mentally ill or disabled people; family members or even an interpreter may be required for people from different ethnic groups, especially if they have a language problem. Information volunteered by the person is classified as subjective, whereas other types of information, such as data from measurement, are objective. The use of objective measures is becoming more common in nursing, partly an outcome of nursing research, for example the use of tools for assessing patients' risk of developing pressure sores and for assessing levels of coma, and levels of pain.

In building up a database for each person, the initial assessment is of great importance although, as has been said, this is only the beginning and not the end of assessing. The first meeting of nurse and patient may be in the person's own home, a nursing home, the health centre, prior to or during admission to hospital (whether as an emergency or from the waiting list).

At whichever location, assessing should ideally be carried out as early as possible in the person's encounter with the health service. As far as hospital is concerned, in reality it is often not possible to collect extensive information within a few hours of admission, so a 'first-stage history' which provides enough information for the nurses to start looking after the patient can be followed as soon as possible by using a more detailed second-stage format. There are, however, some topics about which information must be collected early. Any bleeding or injury would of course be assessed immediately and information about pressure sores or any bruises is essential. It is also necessary for the staff to know of any sensitivities, allergies and any medicines that are currently being taken. All of this information is important to record, whatever the location.

Many employing authorities now provide specific stationery on which the information from nursing assessment is written.

Beginning nurses may be confused by the various names that are used for it: nursing assessment form, patient assessment form, nursing history and patient profile. Whatever the name and format, the objective is to record two different sorts of information: for our purposes, one we call the patient's 'biographical and health data', and the other is 'Activities of Living data' (insofar as they are affected by lifespan, dependence/independence status and the five factors), which are concerned with the individual's usual routines and current problems. We designed suitable forms for recording these two different sorts of data; they are illustrated in Appendix 2.

When the pro forma was first designed, nursing documentation, at least in the UK, was scarcely developed beyond the traditional Kardex system and, indeed, much of the detailed information about a patient was still communicated among nurses by word of mouth at the 'handover' or in the course of day-to-day interaction. In order to help nurses understand how the conceptual thinking of our model could provide a framework for documentation, we introduced into the third edition of *The Elements of Nursing* (1990) a suggested outline for the recording of 'biographical and health data' and 'Activities of Living data', and some refinements have been made since 1990 (Appendix 2).

However, many different approaches to the documentation of patient information are being introduced into healthcare settings. In community-based health care and in hospital settings, there is increasing interest in the development of multiprofessional documentation. Sometimes these are based on clinical packages or clinical guidelines, and sometimes they are specific to the medical diagnosis. On the other hand, some multiprofessional integrated patient records are problem-based; indeed, this approach was first advocated by Weed in 1969. Our model fits well with that approach and nurses may wish to adopt it as the underpinning framework for a multiprofessional documentation system.

In addition, alongside these changes in the approach to documentation, there are current changes in the system of recording. When we first introduced the pro forma, it was universal in the UK for record-keeping to be in written form with records maintained by hand. Now, the computer is taking over and computerized records are increasingly used in healthcare settings, some of them being accessed by both community and hospital personnel.

So, currently, healthcare records are in a transition stage. In some facilities they are uniprofessional, in others multiprofessional. In some they are written/typed records, in others computerized. As far as this monograph is concerned, the pro forma described refers essentially to a uniprofessional record indicating the nursing contribution to the client's healthcare plan. However, provided nurses are clear about the contribution that nursing makes to client/patient care, the data could be adapted for use in a multidisciplinary and/or computerized record. Whatever the approach and form, the following conceptual discussion will still be helpful to nurse learners when documenting the outcome of their professional contact with a client/patient.

Biographical and health data. The person's biographical and health details include obvious items such as name, sex, age, usual place of residence and the person or people to contact when the client requires the assistance of a friend or family member, or when the client's health status is giving cause for concern.

Surname. The custom in Western countries is to use the surname or, in the case of a married woman, the husband's family name, but this is not so in all cultures and nurses may need to seek expert help, firstly to address the person in a manner acceptable to the person, and secondly to be able to retrieve stored data easily according to surname.

Related to surname is the use of the prefix Mr, Mrs, Miss, Ms or other title. Although these titles remain in common use, the increasingly varied social relationships and changing social mores mean that the nurse must be skilful about deciding whether or not it is really necessary to enquire about and/or record a formal title; and whether or not it is necessary to enquire about marital status and other relationships. Of course, the person may volunteer this type of information.

First name. Likewise, it used to be customary to talk about 'Christian' names, but with changing social mores the word 'forename' or 'first name' is now widely used. Increasingly nurses are directed to ask patients/clients what form of address they prefer, as some people use a name other than the one on their birth certificate, and use of the familiar name can help them retain their sense of personal identity.

Use of first names has become more common in social life over the past few decades, and even in working life. In the health service, too, the use of first names between nurses and patients/clients has become more widespread. Originally it was an attempt to create a less formal, more friendly atmosphere, but several research projects have revealed that the use of first names is not always acceptable, especially for the majority of older patients/clients, and particularly when they enter a hospital or nursing home with all the attendant feelings about loss of power, status and independence. On the first contact, it is courteous for the nurse to address adults formally according to the client's cultural norm, and skill is needed to ensure that the client feels sufficiently comfortable to state clearly the preferred form of address. For a vulnerable person who feels ill, worried or distressed, small discourtesies assume for them a major importance.

Age. This information obviously is indicative of stage in the lifespan and is an important consideration in nursing.

Usual place of residence. As well as the person's address, it is becoming more common to record the type of living accommodation, information that is particularly relevant to community nurses on relief duty when visiting people in their own homes. Noting the 'mode of entry' to the house may be necessary information for the community nurse who needs to know how to gain entry when, for example, the person is unable to answer the doorbell. Knowing who resides with the client may also be relevant in certain circumstances.

At times of high unemployment and redundancy, of course, it is salutary to remember that not all people live permanently in a house. There are people who have 'no fixed address'. They may be in 'bed and breakfast' accommodation, or the local authority may provide hostels where homeless people can sleep overnight, or there may be provision for a temporary refuge for 'battered wives', or, especially in larger urban areas, some homeless people may sleep on the streets. The absence of a permanent address, of course, may be culturally determined. In some areas of the world there are nomadic people, and there are 'travelling people' and gypsies. And all too frequently nowadays, there are refugees who are rendered homeless by war or because of major natural disasters.

Contact person and significant others. 'Next of kin' requires to be known for legal purposes and, usually, is the person to be contacted if the patient/client's condition is giving rise to concern. This is pertinent in a hospital setting but is also appropriate if the client is attending a clinic for an invasive investigation (e.g. a gastroenterological procedure); or a day surgery appointment; or in a home setting, for example when the community nurse is tending someone who lives alone, or is elderly, or is vulnerable. The contact person is often in a spouse, parent or child relationship, but with changing social mores an adult may choose to name a partner or friend, and in any case this may be necessary if blood relatives are domiciled abroad.

As well as the named contact person(s), it is sometimes important to know about significant others in terms of the person's social network and sources of support such as relatives, dependants, visitors, helpers and neighbours. In the hospital setting, it may be necessary to record any specific support services being used before admission such as meals-on-wheels or visiting by the community nurse, because on discharge arrangements have to be made for their resumption.

Occupation. This is a useful piece of information. From a health point of view, it may have contributed to the person's current problem, for example an injury sustained at work; in other instances there may be inability to return to former employment, for example when an injury causes paraplegia. Of course, it is well researched that the state of unemployment is not conducive to mental and physical health and well-being.

Religion/beliefs and practices. Religious and other beliefs, and possible accompanying practices, are often very personal and private matters which clients do not wish to discuss. However, relevant information could be recorded if it had implications for nursing interventions associated with the nursing plan.

Recent significant life events or crises. The recording of recent significant life events such as marriage or childbirth may sometimes be relevant, and a recent life crisis such as bereavement may impede recovery. In any event, it is important for the nurse to be aware of, and sympathetic about, any major recent events in a client's life.

Current health problem and reason for contacting the health service. It is useful to know the client's, and when appropriate the family's, perception of the person's current health problem. Asking about the reason for contacting the health service can give an indication of the person's level of understanding of the precipitating factors or, at the other extreme, a lack of knowledge and understanding. When admission to hospital is involved, the reason for admission or referral can be recorded, and also relevant information about the person's diagnosis, past medical history and any allergies. It is usual also to record the address and telephone number of the person's family doctor.

Discharge planning. Making plans for discharge from the healthcare facility acknowledges that, right from the time of entry to the system, it is important to consider the need for health teaching, rehabilitation and discharge planning. If a hospital admission is involved, it is crucial to have adequate and rapid communication with community personnel should supervision be needed following discharge, for example for people who have certain mental illnesses, or for elderly people who are discharged from acute wards.

This outline gives some idea of the type of information that might be collected at an initial assessment. These biographical and health data should be available to all nursing staff whether the person's stay in the health service is short or long term.

Assessing ALs. The second part of assessing focuses on the person's ALs: the individual's usual routines and current problems. Use of the ALs for assessment is central to our model of nursing and each of the person's relevant ALs is assessed in the context of the other concepts of the model—lifespan, dependence/independence status, the five factors, and therefore individuality in living (as brief examples, assessing related to three of the 12 ALs is given in Appendix 3).

Data collected in the context of the five influencing factors outline each person in his or her entirety. Those who will nurse the person need to know about usual routines—importantly what the person can and cannot do independently—and whether or not there are any problems or discomforts associated with any AL; if so, whether these have been experienced previously and, if this is the case, how they have been coped with.

The form (Appendix 2) on which AL assessment information is recorded is deliberately without ruled spaces for each AL so that the nurse can use the space to best advantage for each particular client/patient, ordering the data in terms of the most problematic ALs first or whatever seems the most appropriate order in the circumstances and not necessarily commenting on each AL if such information is not relevant to the current episode. A few general comments will, however, be made about each AL.

- *Assessing ability to maintain a safe environment* is of particular importance if the person is physically or mentally disabled or has a learning impairment. The nurse needs to know whether or not the person appreciates the dangers in the environment and knows how to prevent accidents. Assessing the level of safety in the home is an important responsibility of the nurse who visits elderly people or families with young children.

- *Assessing communicating skills* is necessary in order to discover the person's level of communication and this is important whether in the home, health centre or hospital; indeed, any information given or received about any of the other ALs is via the medium of the AL of communicating. It is very important for nurses who have an extensive technical vocabulary to remember that not all people will be familiar with nursing and medical terms, however ordinary or straightforward they seem to staff.

The nurse should observe whether the person is reticent or forthcoming when talking about home and health problems. It is sometimes possible to discern from the conversation whether the person is gregarious by nature or shy, and it may be necessary to gather specific information about one of the sensory organs if the nurse suspects a deficiency or dysfunction which is affecting the person's AL of communicating. Finally, when assessing this AL, any general information about the person's pain should be sought and recorded. The rationale for linking pain with the AL of communicating is based on the fact that pain is a subjective experience; its presence and degree is communicated to us by the person's verbal and non-verbal behaviour. Additional data about pain which affects specific ALs (e.g. abdominal pain affecting the AL of eating and drinking) can be recorded at that AL.

The ability to communicate is essential, obviously, if any recommended procedures require 'informed consent'.

- *Assessing breathing* may involve counting the number of respirations per minute. For the majority of people, however, it is simply a case of the nurse noting whether there is an apparent breathing difficulty and asking if they have a problem with a cough or breathlessness. In turn, this may offer an opportunity to discover whether or not the person smokes and, if so, how much. The nurse should attempt to discover the person's perception of the multiple ill-effects of smoking and whether or not help with giving up or reducing the habit of smoking would be welcomed.

More detailed assessment of breathing is necessary when a patient is unconscious, still under the effects of an anaesthetic, or suffering from a disease affecting the cardiopulmonary system. It should be noted that information about haemorrhage (other than bleeding related to a specific AL; e.g. vaginal bleeding would pertain to the AL of expressing sexuality) should be recorded under the AL of breathing on the basis that, in our model, the cardiopulmonary system is allocated to this AL.

• *Assessing eating and drinking routines* is relatively easy because most people enjoy talking about this AL. When nursing underweight and overweight people it is especially important to talk with them about what they eat, as well as when and how much. Nurses will need information about how people with certain disabilities manage this activity. When the person complains of discomfort associated with eating or drinking, more specific assessment will be required.

• *Assessing a person's eliminating habits* is a nursing function even though admission to the healthcare system may not have been associated with bowel or urinary dysfunction. But there may well be a persistent problem with, for example, constipation and this may be elicited from the assessment. Many people find it embarrassing to talk about elimination and the nurse needs to broach the topic with sensitivity and phrase the questions carefully and clearly to avoid embarrassment yet elicit information.

• *Assessing personal cleansing habits and dressing* is possible by observing the result of these activities; ill-cared-for clothes may be an indication of financial hardship or a lack of self-esteem which can characterize exhaustion or mental illness. The nurse may discover unhygienic practices, for example related to cleaning teeth, or related to lack of handwashing after visiting the toilet. With this knowledge the nurse can plan to include relevant teaching in the nursing plan. It should be noted that assessment of the AL of personal cleansing and dressing should include an assessment of the patient's skin status (including signs of bruising which could be the result of physical abuse) and an assessment of the person's risk of developing pressure sores if appropriate. The rationale for including this here is on the basis that biologically, in our model, the integumentary system is allocated to this AL.

• *Assessing control of body temperature* often involves taking the person's temperature whether at home, in the clinic or in hospital, and regular measurement may become necessary if the person is suffering from pyrexia or hypothermia. There are other ways of assessing this AL: observation may reveal flushing of the skin, excessive perspiration, the presence of goose flesh, shivering, and excessively hot or cold hands and/or feet.

• *Assessing mobilizing* may involve only observing that the person does not appear to have any problems. But later observation or discussion might reveal, for example, stiffness of the joints on rising after sleep, a common occurrence for the older person. People who have persistent back pain often adopt a characteristic posture to minimize low back movement. Other mobilizing problems are usually self-evident and nurses need to know how the person copes with them; detailed information should be obtained on this from physically disabled people so that nursing can be planned to enable maximum independence to be retained, including continuing use of mobilizing aids.

• *Assessing working and playing routines* is an essential part of an initial overall patient assessment. By the way the person talks about these activities, the nurse will gather what is considered challenging and what is boring or stressful. The physical conditions at the person's place of work may have contributed to the accident or illness which has necessitated attendance at the clinic or admission to hospital. On the other hand, difficulty in social relationships because of personality problems or mental illness may be revealed or suspected, and difficulties inherent in enforced unemployment would be important to know about for people in that situation.

• *Assessing the AL of expressing sexuality* involves observing how people express their gender in a general way, for example in mode of dress, use of cosmetics and so on. Specific assessment is not usually necessary or appropriate unless the person's problems or potential problems are somehow associated with sexuality, or sex and reproduction; most people find it embarrassing to talk with strangers about this private AL. However, the observant nurse will perceive cues which are expressions of sexuality, or indicators of anxieties related to the AL of expressing sexuality. With sensitivity the nurse can create an atmosphere in which people feel able to discuss sex-related problems and diseases, if appropriate, and a detailed assessment may become necessary in certain circumstances.

• *Assessing sleeping routines* at an early stage is important so that nurses have information on which to base nursing activities aimed at promoting sleep. People do not usually contact health personnel specifically because of a sleep problem as such, but adequate sleep is important for health, whatever the reason for coming into contact with the health service, and promotion of sleep requires knowledge of the person's usual routines and use of medication, if any.

● *Assessing the needs of the dying* is a very important role of the nurse in the community as well as in hospitals, nursing homes and hospices. Although we included the AL of dying in our list of 12 ALs, 'assessing' becomes essential only when the diagnosis and prognosis indicate that the person's death is probable in the immediate or near future. However, constant sensitivity and acute observation are necessary to recognize whether or not the person wants to talk about the many aspects associated with death, dying and bereavement—even a healthy young mother with a healthy baby may have concerns about potential cot death.

Assessing is not a once-only activity and additional data will be collected as the nurses have further opportunity to observe people and talk with them in the course of their nursing. Whether additional data are obtained and recorded on a daily basis or less frequently will depend on factors such as the person's condition, length of stay in hospital, nursing home, hospice, or frequency of visits in the case of a person at home or attending a clinic.

Equally, the amount and type of information collected about the ALs will vary according to different circumstances and, in some, information about all of the ALs may not be relevant. Assessing, therefore, is not a rigid routine carried out at a particular time and in a set pattern; it is an ongoing activity and one that requires to be tailored to the circumstances of the individual person.

Assessing is just as applicable to people who are in the health-care system for surveillance or maintenance of health as for those who are in hospital for investigation and/or treatment of illness. Some nurses think that the identification of patients' problems is not applicable to health maintenance and promotion, but in healthy living the aim is to avoid potential problems from becoming actual ones, and the process of identifying potential problems with the ALs is the same as that involved in the identification of actual problems.

Whatever the health or illness status, while collecting information about the person's ALs the nurse will necessarily take account of the stage on the lifespan, one of the components of the model. There is a reminder on our proforma (Appendix 2) to consider the person's 'previous routines' and it is necessary to remember that these will have been fashioned by biological, psychological, sociocultural, environmental and politicoeconomic factors—another component of the model. The nurse is reminded of the dependence/independence continuum of the model by the heading 'what can/cannot be done independently'. And there is a prompt 'previous coping mechanisms' to remind the nurse that, if there are problems or discomforts with any of the ALs, enquiry should be made about how these have been coped with.

In summary, then, the objective in collecting information about the ALs is to discover:

- previous routines
- what the person can do independently
- what the person cannot do independently
- previous coping behaviours
- what problems the person has, both actual and potential, with relevant ALs.

Identifying the individual's problems. Identifying the person's problems is the final activity of the assessing phase of the process of nursing. As stated earlier, the nurse's role is to enable the patient/client to prevent, alleviate or solve, or cope positively with problems (actual or potential) related to the ALs. In many cases, the presence of *actual* problems (such as pain, bleeding, anorexia, pyrexia, acute depression, learning disability) may be obvious to the person and often is obvious to the nurse. But it has to be remembered that there may be a 'nurse-perceived problem' of which the patient is not aware (raised blood pressure being an obvious example), or a 'patient-perceived problem' (such as a particular worry or obsessive behaviour or suicidal tendencies) of which the nurse is not immediately aware. Being alert to these possibilities will ensure that they are explored in the course of assessment.

When it comes to identifying *potential* problems, the nurse's greater knowledge of factors that predispose to ill-health, and are complications of illness and treatment, makes it possible to collect information that the person may not volunteer without prompting. It is the concept of potential problems that also highlights the aspects of nursing which are concerned with the maintenance and promotion of health.

A statement of the person's problems, as ascertained from the nursing assessment, is increasingly being referred to as 'a nursing diagnosis'. A reluctance to use this term in nursing, at least in the UK, may be for the reason that 'diagnosis' is traditionally the doctor's role. But, in fact, a nursing diagnosis is a description of the problems that people experience with ALs, whereas the medical diagnosis is usually concerned with pathological changes. In fact, a person with one medical diagnosis may have several nursing diagnoses.

In recent years, considerable work has been undertaken, particularly in North America, to develop a method of classifying nursing diagnoses—what we term 'problems'. Currently, a panel working with the International Council of Nurses (ICN) has commenced collating information and ideas from its Member Associations around the world with the aim of producing an international classification of nursing practices; the objective is to provide a 'common language' which will promote shared understanding among nurses worldwide. The related ICN publications (1996, 1999) define nursing diagnoses as 'the description given by nurses to phenomena which are the focus for nursing intervention'. It is a complex classification intended for computer use and will be an ongoing exercise.

The idea of a patient/client's problems with ALs is still relevant although, in time, its terminology may need to be linked with other classifications. The pro forma which we prepared for *The Elements of Nursing* (Appendix 2) provides space for each identified problem, specified as 'actual' or as 'potential' by noting '(p)' against the latter.

Having undertaken an adequate assessment, all that remains before proceeding with planning is to decide on the relative priority among the problems. It hardly needs to be said that life-threatening and health-threatening problems take precedence over other less immediate or less important problems and, among these, the priority will be decided in collaboration with the person and, if appropriate, with the family. The person's priority may not always be the same as the nurse's, and this must be taken into account for it will affect motivation and cooperation. The priority among problems can be indicated on the form by arranging the problems in order or, alternatively, numbering their priority.

Planning

The second phase of the process of nursing is planning, and it reflects our definition of nursing. The objective of the plan is:

- to prevent identified potential problems with any of the ALs from becoming actual ones
- to solve identified actual problems
- where possible, to alleviate those that cannot be solved
- to help the person cope positively with those problems that cannot be alleviated or solved
- to prevent recurrence of a treated problem
- to help the person to be as comfortable and pain-free as possible when death is inevitable.

Setting goals. To achieve this, a goal has to be set for each actual and potential problem (in collaboration with the person whenever possible, and perhaps with the family) with a distinction made between short-term and long-term goals. Instead of the word 'goals' some nurses prefer 'objectives' or 'patient outcomes' or 'desired outcomes'; it is a matter of preference.

Goals should be achievable within a person's individual circumstances, otherwise there is the danger of disheartenment. Whenever possible, goals should be stated in terms of outcomes that are able to be observed, measured or tested so that their subsequent evaluation can be accomplished. Whenever feasible, a time or date should be specified alongside a goal to indicate when evaluation should be undertaken. So the nurse (along with the person, when relevant) sets a goal and estimates when it might be achieved, just as the traveller decides on a destination and, according to the mode of travel, estimates the time of arrival. But, it needs to be said, such travelling is considerably less complicated and more certain than nursing.

Preparing a nursing plan. Before nursing plans can be written, or put into a computer, account has to be taken of existing resources which in a nursing context may be equipment, personnel and physical environment; available support services may have to be considered when a person is being nursed at home. Possible alternative nursing interventions may be determined by the availability of resources and influenced by the person's expressed preferences.

A plan is then made of all the proposed nursing interventions to achieve the goals, stated in sufficient detail so that any other nurse, on reading it, would be aware of the plan of nursing. There is no argument against a written or computerized plan being essential since no one nurse can be on duty throughout the 24 hours. Social changes such as decreased working hours, and an increase in both annual leave and use of part-time staff, have made it essential for nurses to develop the skill of communicating with colleagues by recording adequate nursing plans. If such social trends continue, it may well be that the nursing plan will assume even greater importance as a means of communication between nurses. And, furthermore, assessing a person and recording a nursing plan helps the nurse to know the person, which aids the establishment of a satisfactory nurse–patient relationship, an important dimension of the nursing contribution to a person's health care.

The nursing plan, which is part of the pro forma for use with the model, is shown in Appendix 2. There is a section for noting nurse-initiated interventions (i.e. those derived from problems with ALs) and another section which is for medically prescribed interventions (e.g. medical prescriptions for pain management). Explanation of these sections of the nursing plan is provided below.

Nursing plan related to ALs. The nursing plan on page three of our document (Appendix 2) is related to the ALs and it forms the right side of the double fold. This positioning is deliberate so that the problems, both actual and potential, identified at the initial assessment do not need to be written again. Opposite the problems the goals are written, together with the 'nurse-initiated interventions' to achieve these, and there is a column in which to record the result of 'evaluation'.

The nursing plan may have nursing interventions at an AL even although there is not a specific problem stated, for example when the person does not have a problem with the AL of personal cleansing and dressing but has a particular preference for a shower rather than a bath. Noting this fact will alert nurses reading the plan to the person's preference and deter them from initiating an alternative form of intervention. Similarly, a disabled person may not have a problem as such with the AL of mobilizing as long as aids that are relied on remain available; noting details of the person's requirements for 'aided independence' will avoid unnecessary dependence on the nursing staff as well as frustration for the person.

The nursing plan is just that: a *plan* which tells nurses what to do and when. Extra information should be recorded only:

- when a goal or desired outcome has been achieved
- when the nursing intervention has to be changed to achieve the already set goal
- when, for any reason, the goal has to be modified
- when the date for evaluation has changed
- if the person develops other problems.

Other day-to-day information about the person should be recorded in the patient's nursing notes, and pro formas for these kinds of recordings are usually devised locally.

Nursing plan derived from medical or other prescription. We have discussed so far the nurse-initiated nursing interventions related to ALs, but clearly there are nursing interventions that are derived directly from medical prescription and, increasingly, from the prescriptions of other members of the healthcare team such as the dietitian or physiotherapist. Although some such prescriptions may be charted separately (e.g. prescribed drugs on the person's medicine chart), others are not, and it was for this reason that we decided to add this fourth page to the nursing pro forma.

Inclusion of these nursing interventions does not mean a return to the 'medical model', a term, incidentally, that does not appear in the medical literature. Nursing is a collaborative activity and it irrefutably includes interventions arising from medical prescription, but thereafter they are nursing interventions and in the domain of our model as helping to solve or alleviate people's problems.

At the bottom of this part of the nursing plan is a space for 'other notes'. The information that could be recorded here might be about the time and place of clinic appointments; arrangements for transport to and from these clinics; and particulars about the loan of equipment, such as a walking frame for the person to use at home. These examples alert the nurse to the fact that planning is necessary for the person's discharge from the health service facility. Discharge planning starts at the initial assessment, as acknowledged on our suggested form for biographical and health data (Appendix 2). However, there is no constraint on the type of relevant information that nurses may record in the space for 'other notes' and on pages 5 and 6 of the pro forma.

Summarizing the planning phase of the process: it involves producing a nursing plan that contains the following information:

- stated goals or desired outcomes for each problem
- a date on which the goals are expected to be achieved
- the nursing interventions (and patient participation) to achieve the goals.

The objective of the nursing plan is to provide the information on which systematic, individualized nursing can be based and implemented by any nurse; when appropriate, the information can be incorporated in a multidisciplinary plan using a computerized record.

Implementing the nursing plan

Implementing the plan of nursing is the third phase of the process of nursing. Traditionally, nursing has been associated with 'doing', so nurses have little difficulty in knowing how to go about this phase of the process. It is being recognized increasingly, however, that it is both helpful and necessary for nurses to make explicit the thinking and decision-making which underlie and explain the nursing interventions that they carry out.

Activities that could be described as 'nursing interventions' are many and varied. For any one person it is likely that the number and range of nursing activities carried out will far exceed those specifically listed in the nursing plan. It is likely that the plan will include all the essential and important 'main' interventions but, alongside carrying out these particular, specified activities, the nurse will be doing many other things as well—what Meleis (1997) calls 'the dailiness of nurses' work'.

In carrying out nursing interventions, the nurse draws on an amalgam of skills—from listening, talking and observing to helping and, perhaps, deliberately not helping—in their contact with the person over time. It may be that some of the 'unplanned' or apparently 'unimportant' interventions of this kind seem to merit recording. The pro forma for use with the model does not contain a section for these purposes and we suggest the use of a separate sheet or document which could be called 'patient's nursing notes'. These would contain information supplementary to the patient assessment form and nursing plan. Such information could be helpful for purposes of evaluating nursing intervention, both ongoing and summative.

Evaluating

It is difficult to justify planning and implementing nursing interventions if the outcome cannot be shown to have benefited the recipients in some way. Hence, the fourth phase of the process of nursing—evaluating—is crucial and, in turn, provides a basis for ongoing assessment and planning as the person's circumstances and problems change.

The evaluating phase of the process initially has caused considerable difficulties for nurses. This is not surprising because evaluation is an extremely difficult and complex matter, and this is true not only in respect of nursing. Put simply, the objective of evaluating is to find out whether or not (or to what extent) the goals that were set have been (or are being) achieved. In this sense, evaluation is of the type known as 'outcome evaluation'. The skills used in evaluating are essentially similar to those used in assessing: observing, questioning, examining, testing and measuring. Whereas they are used in assessing to provide baseline data, in evaluating they are used to discover whether or not the set goals are being or have been achieved: in other words, evaluating involves comparison against an objective.

Goal achievement in effect renders the nursing intervention redundant. However, it may be necessary to ask the question: 'Was the goal set too low? and a reconsideration of the original goal setting might answer this question. In the absence of successful goal achievement the nurse might ask:

- Is it partially achieved and is more information needed before reconsidering whether or not to continue or adapt the intervention?
- Is the problem unchanged or static, and should the nursing intervention be changed or stopped?
- Is there a worsening of the problem and should the goal and the planned nursing intervention be reviewed?
- Was the goal incorrectly stated or inappropriate?
- Does the goal require intervention(s) from other members of the healthcare team?

The last question recognizes that the contribution by other health workers in a multidisciplinary team inevitably influences and interacts with their own intervention and, indeed, it is seldom possible to isolate the nursing intervention and, therefore, directly and unequivocally link the 'outcome' with 'input'. Thus, the evaluating phase of the nursing process is beset with complexities and an important challenge for the future in nursing will be to improve and extend our evaluation skills.

We advocate documentation in process format, illustrated in Figure 3.7. The objective when using the phases of the process is to individualize nursing. Individualizing is a dynamic process and Figure 3.8 illustrates this, using our model of nursing as a conceptual framework.

As a postscript, conceptualizing nursing in the way proposed in this chapter, and documenting it in process format with the objective of individualizing nursing, need not be the only goal. Documentation can give greater job satisfaction; nurses do not personally work on a 24-hour rota so on return to duty they can read about what has happened in their absence thereby contributing a sense of continuity and participation; indeed, it is the record (written or computerized) that provides evidence of continuity. Documents can be so worded that they:

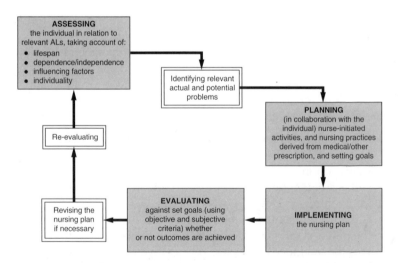

Figure 3.8 Individualizing nursing as a dynamic process using the Roper-Logan-Tierney model of nursing as a conceptual framework.

- are a part of a monitoring programme related to the quality of nursing service
- provide factual information to managers when, because of staff shortages, items in the 'planned nursing' had to be omitted
- provide factual information to managers when a second-best nursing intervention had to be planned because of lack of resources
- provide information that can be used in defence of patients' complaints in a legal context
- help nurses to describe nursing's contribution to the total healthcare programme, particularly important when submitting an application for adequate financial resources
- provide substantiation for adequate remuneration for nursing personnel
- contribute to a database for research in nursing.

In conclusion, it must be stated that the preceding text advocates documentation of nursing practice and emphasizes the need for accuracy and quality in preparing such records. Inherent in record-keeping, of course, are the responsibilities of confidentiality, accountability and personal liability, and with the increasing use of computerized records—and the related Data Protection Acts—these responsibilities are, in fact, even more onerous. For tomorrow's nurses, 'embracing the future' holds many challenges.

REFERENCES

Charatan F 1994 Psychiatrists in US put religion in diagnostic manual. British Medical Journal 308(6931):740

Fawcett J 1995 Analysis and evaluation of conceptual models of nursing, 3rd edn. F A Davis, Philadelphia

Henderson V 1969 The basic principles of nursing care. International Council of Nurses, Geneva

International Council of Nurses 1996 The international classification for nursing practice: a unifying framework. The alpha version. ICN, Geneva

International Council of Nurses 1999 The international classification for nursing practice: a unifying framework. The beta version. ICN, Geneva

Meleis A 1997 Theoretical nursing: development and progress, 3rd edn. J B Lippincott, Philadelphia

Richards A 1998 Partnership with patients. British Medical Journal 316(10):85

Roper N 1976 Clinical experience in nurse education. Churchill Livingstone, Edinburgh

United Nations Population Fund 1999 Six billion: a time for choice; the state of the world population. UN, New York

Weed L L 1969 Medical records, medical education and patient care—the problem-orientated record as a basic tool. Case Western Reserve University Press, Cleveland, Ohio

4

Assessment of the model

In the opening chapter of this monograph, the background to the development of the Roper-Logan-Tierney model of nursing was outlined and in the ensuing chapters the model of living and the model of nursing were described. As explained, the model was refined progressively in each of the four editions of *The Elements of Nursing* over the period from 1980 to 1996. The beginnings of the model, however, date back to the early 1970s and so, at the time of writing this text—as the 1990s draw to a close—our model has been under ongoing development for almost three decades. Now, on the threshold of a new millennium, and in an era of unprecedented speed of change in healthcare systems and across society at large, it is interesting to attempt to make some assessment of the contribution of this model—and of nursing models in

---

This chapter draws on a paper presented by Alison Tierney at the First International Nursing Theory Conference held in Germany in April 1997 which, in turn, was subsequently developed into a paper published as Tierney A J 1998 Nursing models: extant or extinct? Journal of Advanced Nursing 28(1): 77–85.

general—to the development of nursing over the latter half of the twentieth century and in anticipation of the challenges for nursing worldwide as we enter the twenty-first century.

The value of nursing models

Over the past decade, the benefits (and disbenefits) of nursing models have been discussed and debated at some length, sometimes with considerable emotion. In the UK—the home of the Roper-Logan-Tierney model—there is no doubt that, from the outset, the very idea of nursing models was dismissed outright in some circles. It could be argued that the early critics of models were simply antithetical to any form of development that appeared to be 'academic' in nature, and so nursing models were summarily dismissed as mere 'armchair theorizing'. In contrast, more recent critiques of models which can be found in the nursing literature can be seen to represent more serious contributions to a more informed debate, worldwide, about ways in which 'the nature of nursing' can be conceptualized. Some of the writing about models has focused narrowly on the particular question of their *practical* utility (Kenny 1993, Luker 1988) but, increasingly, the value of models is also being debated in the overall context of knowledge-building in nursing. Such debates are challenging and helpful in raising important questions about lines of enquiry for the advancement of nursing knowledge and practice.

Draper's (1990) paper is an example of the more detailed and analytic writing about 'nursing theory' that began to emanate from the UK in the 1990s. However, on the specific question of the perceived value of nursing models, Draper concluded that, at least in the UK, there had been a generally uncritical adoption of American frameworks and little evident impact of models on clinical nursing. Cash (1990) scrutinized some of these conceptual frameworks more closely and concluded that 'what we have (in nursing models) is nursing being so generally defined that it loses its identity'; indeed, he went as far as to propose that 'the search for such a scheme should be removed from the agenda of nurse thinkers'.

The views of Cash (1990) and Draper (1990) are not isolated criticisms. Others also have suggested that nursing models may have been positively unhelpful to knowledge-building in nursing by inhibiting alternative, more fruitful, lines of theory development (Chalmers et al 1990). And Biley (1992), while acknowledging that nursing models may have been 'an essential step' in the initial theoretical development of nursing, argued strongly that they now had become redundant in practice, and she proposed that 'the intuitive' must replace 'the empirical' as the primary route to theory-building for nursing practice. These arguments epitomize the increasing polarization in nursing between adherents to different schools of theoretical thinking.

A growing polarization of views has been apparent in the North American context for even longer than in the UK, and Reed's (1995) paper provides a skilful analysis of the tensions there between modernist (i.e. essentially positivist) and post-modernist perspectives, both in general terms and, specifically, in relation to nursing models. 'In the modernist era', Reed observes, 'these models were regarded as ideas to be revered, preserved, unaltered, and used in their entirety'. Now, in the 1990s, she notes, nursing models are being disparaged on grounds that nursing 'has matured beyond needing the conceptual models for knowledge development and practice'. Reed envisages the possibility of an era beyond post-modernism in which theoretical thinking in nursing adopts an 'open philosophy' and embraces various forms of theorizing and, in that scenario, Reed argues that there is a continuing role for nursing models.

The role of nursing models

What, then, is the role of nursing models? This question really has been answered already in the opening chapter of this monograph. As explained there, nursing models seemed, at least to the early American nurse theorists, to provide a fruitful way of beginning to think theoretically about nursing: to provide a way of attempting to answer that elusive question: 'What is nursing?'. Reflect again on Reilly's (1975) explanation of what the proponents of the early nursing models were actually doing. She stated:

We all have a private image (concept) of nursing practice. In turn, this private image influences our interpretation of data, our decisions, and our actions. But can a discipline continue to develop when its members hold so many differing private images? The proponents of conceptual models of practice are seeking to make us aware of these private images, so that we can begin to identify commonalities in our perceptions of the nature of practice and move towards a well-ordered concept.

Note that Reilly refers to 'concept' in the singular. The idea that a single, unified model of nursing might emerge—one 'world view' of the discipline—was encouraged initially by some nurse theorists (e.g. Riehl & Roy 1980). But the fact that different models have survived over time has to be interpreted as implying that there is perceived value in (or at least tolerance of) the coexistence of various conceptual frameworks in nursing, rather than any overriding demand for just one.

Instead, there have been efforts to highlight the similarities among coexisting frameworks, and in the 1980s these were encapsulated in the identification of four concepts—'person', 'environment', 'health' and 'nursing'—which, together, make up what Fawcett (1984) described as nursing's 'metaparadigm'. Although this conceptualization has been widely used, more recently Meleis & Trangenstein (1994) have argued that the very varied interpretation of the metaparadigm concepts, and the paucity in their systematic development over time, now raises questions about their utility in providing the discipline of nursing with a coherent definition and any clear direction for knowledge development. So where does this place nursing models now?

The place (and nature) of nursing models

One of the problems in trying to discuss the place of nursing models in the changing landscape of nursing theory is that much of the theoretical debate in nursing has been dogged by terminological imprecision and confusion. Nursing models have been variously referred to as philosophies, conceptual frameworks, paradigms, theories, grand theories and metatheories. Fawcett (1995) continues to advocate the term 'conceptual models of nursing' and her definition, which was introduced early in this text, is helpful to look at again for purposes of the present discussion:

Conceptual models are made up of concepts, which are words describing mental images of phenomena, and propositions, which are statements expressing the relations between concepts. A conceptual model, therefore, is designed as a set of concepts and the statements that integrate them into a meaningful configuration. (Fawcett 1984)

Fawcett has emphasized consistently that a conceptual model is not a theory. In contrast, Meleis (1997) takes a more liberal view of the term 'theory', extending it to embrace conceptual frameworks and rejecting the narrow view of theory as a term reserved only for research-verified propositions. However, Fawcett~ insistence on differentiating between models and theories can be helpful. Her distinction is in terms of the level of abstraction within what she refers to as 'the structural hierarchy' of knowledge (Fawcett 1995). Theories, according to this schema, sit lower down the ladder of abstraction than models. A model is, in Fawcett's terms, 'a highly abstract system of global concepts' and, while models can generate theory, by this analysis they are not theory in their own right.

Fawcett (1992, 1995) considers that at least seven different frameworks which comply with the definition of a conceptual model (as she has defined it) are used in contemporary nursing practice:

1. Dorothy Johnson's Behavioral System Model
2. Imogene King's Systems Framework
3. Myra Levine's Conservation Model
4. Betty Neuman's Systems Model
5. Dorothea Orem's Self-Care Framework
6. Martha Rogers' Science of Unitary Human Beings
7. Callista Roy's Adaptation Model.

Typically, American theory writers—Fawcett included—have not acknowledged nursing models that originate outside North America; hence the Roper-Logan-Tierney model of nursing is not included in this list. An important issue in assessing our model, therefore, is to determine whether or not it is a *true* nursing model: in other words, does the Roper-Logan-Tierney model of nursing comply with Fawcett's definition of a conceptual framework?

Is the Roper-Logan-Tierney model a *true* nursing model?

In considering this question, it is important to bear in mind that Fawcett's first text on conceptual models was not published until 1984, and Meleis's seminal book on theoretical nursing first appeared in 1985; so we had almost no 'nursing theory' literature of a general kind to draw on when first working on our model in the 1970s.

We did acquaint ourselves with the first of the models being produced in North America (e.g. Orem 1971, Rogers 1970, Roy

1970) because we knew of these developments from Win Logan's contacts with the United States and Nancy Roper's discovery, in the course of writing her MPhil thesis, of the publication on 'Concept formalization in nursing' from the Nursing Development Conference Group (1973). Theoretical literature of that kind, however, was rare in British nursing libraries in the 1970s. And, of course, as acknowledged, we were influenced strongly by Virginia Henderson's enunciation of the basic principles of nursing care, first published in 1960 (Henderson 1960). That work, however, was not presented in the form of a nursing model per se, and the early models that we did examine gave little guidance about the principles or processes of conceptualization that go into the construction of a model. Indeed, we would have to confess to having found some of the American models quite difficult to understand!

The basis of our own model, then, lay not in 'nursing theory' but instead, as explained in Chapter 1 (p. 9), the basic ideas in the Roper-Logan-Tierney model evolved from the research project on clinical experience in nurse education which had been undertaken by Nancy Roper at the start of the 1970s (Roper 1976a, 1976b, 1979). *The Elements of Nursing* was not written primarily as a contribution to the theoretical nursing literature but, as explained, it was intended primarily for *educational* purposes and, specifically, with the objective of presenting an introductory nursing textbook within a conceptual framework in order to 'assist learners to develop a way of thinking about nursing' across the boundaries of different patient/client groups and different healthcare settings.

Beyond that, of course, we saw potential for the model to provide practising nurses with a framework to assist their use of the nursing process which, at the time, was fast gaining ground in British nursing but, without a conceptual framework, nurses were having difficulty in seeing how to operationalize 'the process' in practice. And we certainly saw the model as a framework that could help to accelerate the shift in British nursing away from its traditionally strong adherence to the *medical* model. Thus, as explained, the Roper-Logan-Tierney model of nursing was focused deliberately on the *independent* (i.e. nurse-initiated) aspects of nursing, although not ignoring the *dependent* (i.e. medically prescribed) functions of nurses and the *interdependent* (i.e. interdisciplinary) activities in which nurses engage.

The emergent model—the Roper-Logan-Tierney model of nursing—has been described in this monograph. Were we—are we—justified in labelling it as a *nursing model*? Is it a *true* nursing model?

The central tenet of Fawcett's (1984) definition of a conceptual model is that it should comprise 'a set of concepts and the statements that integrate them into a meaningful configuration'. In a slightly earlier definition, Riehl & Roy (1980) placed similar emphasis on the idea that a nursing model must be 'systematically constructed' and centred around a 'logically related set of concepts'. Obviously the definitive assessment of whether or not the Roper-Logan-Tierney model fulfils these fundamental principles of conceptualization must be left to readers and critics to decide, but we argue that our model does meet these basic *conceptual* requirements.

The 'set of concepts' that make up the Roper-Logan-Tierney model are the five 'components' of the model, as have been described in the preceding chapters, namely:

- Activities of Living (ALs)
- Lifespan
- Dependence/independence continuum
- Factors influencing ALs
- Individualizing nursing (based on individuality in living).

These concepts are 'logically related' (Riehl & Roy 1980); for example, the links between ALs and lifespan, and between lifespan and the dependence/independence continuum, have been highlighted repeatedly in the previous two chapters. Furthermore, the five concepts in the model can be seen to be integrated into a 'meaningful configuration' (Fawcett 1984). While Figure 4.1 provides a simple way of depicting the overall configuration of the Roper-Logan-Tierney model, it is of course only by studying the accompanying text that readers can gain insight to the relationships between and among the component parts of the model, and gain an understanding of the model as a whole and the values and assumptions that underpin both the parts and the whole. The importance of studying the text attached to this (and any) nursing model cannot be overstated.

It is only from the text, for example, that the model of nursing can be understood as having been based, from the outset, on a model of living. The rationale for linking 'nursing' with 'living'

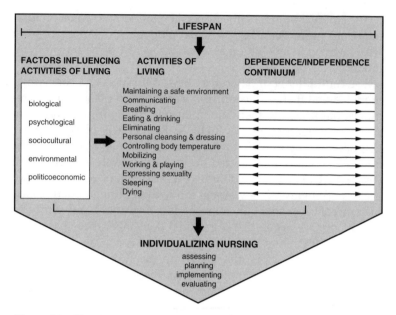

Figure 4.1 The Roper-Logan-Tierney model of nursing.

reflected our growing awareness that people's health and ill-health are inextricably linked with lifestyle and, further, that people's need for nursing is usually only short lived and, therefore, minimal disruption of their established lifestyle should be a primary goal of nursing. This may not seem like avant garde thinking nowadays, but it was a progressive view of nursing in the UK in the early 1970s. And, interestingly, it is a view of nursing—and of patients/clients—that has gained momentum over the intervening years and fits well with contemporary developments in health care as a whole and with the likely future trends.

In both models (i.e. model of living and model of nursing) the focus—the pivotal concept—is described in terms of the *Activities of Living*, this being our chosen device (as explained) for conceptualizing the complex process of 'living'. The 12 ALs are shown at the centre of the diagram of the model (Fig. 4.1) in order to emphasize the centrality of this concept, both to 'living' and to 'nursing'. And, in turn, the way in which we define nursing is congruent with this conceptualization: namely, that nursing is centred on 'helping people to prevent, alleviate, solve or cope with problems (actual or potential) with their Activities of Living'

(Roper et al 1996, p. 35). Patients' problems with the ALs were construed, as clearly included in our definition, as being both *actual* and *potential*, thus enabling the model to place as much emphasis on prevention and health promotion as on helping patients with existing problems. All of these aspects of the model have been highlighted and discussed in the previous chapters. Reiteration here is for purposes of re-focusing attention on the *conceptualization* that underpins our model for purposes of assessing whether or not the Roper-Logan-Tierney model of nursing can be said to fulfil the basic requirements of a nursing model. We would argue that our model does contain all the ingredients that Fawcett (1984, 1995) identified: namely, a clear 'set of concepts' and a clear explanation of how these are integrated into 'a meaningful configuration'.

Literature on the model

Although the description of the Roper-Logan-Tierney model presented in this monograph will provide readers with the most recent version of the model, a more detailed understanding of the model and its development over time can be accessed by studying the four editions of *The Elements of Nursing* (Roper et al 1980, 1985, 1990, 1996). The changes that have been made to the model over time, although summarized in Appendix 1 (pp. 171–178), can be fully appreciated only by examining the previous accounts of the model in detail. Other primary sources of literature on the Roper-Logan-Tierney model (see references shown under Roper et al) include the texts published in 1981 and 1983, one of which illustrated use of the initial version of the model with the nursing process while the other utilized the model in various practice settings; a series of articles in *Nursing Mirror* in 1983; and book chapters in Kershaw & Salvage (1986) and, more recently, in American texts by Hinton-Walker & Neuman (1997) and Marriner Tomey & Alligood (1998).

Secondary sources include numerous articles in nursing journals which refer to our model (a selection of these will be referred to later); chapters on the Roper-Logan-Tierney model in various textbooks on nursing models (e.g. Aggleton & Chalmers 1986, 2000, Fraser 1990, 1996, Pearson & Vaughan 1986, 1996); and also a book based on our model by Newton (1992). Of course, secondary sources that predate the most recent primary source of

information about the model (now this monograph) are, by definition, out of date and failure to draw on the most recent version
of the Roper-Logan-Tierney model has been, regrettably, a not
uncommon feature of the secondary literature. It is, of course, that
literature which allows an assessment of the model to be based
not just on our own claims and reflections but also, importantly,
on the observations and criticisms of others who have no personal investment in the model.

Impact of the model

There is no doubt that, in the UK and elsewhere in Europe, the
Roper-Logan-Tierney model has become very widely known over
the years and, in response to demand, *The Elements of Nursing*
has been translated from English into eight other languages to
date (Dutch, Estonian, Finnish, German, Italian, Lithuanian,
Portuguese and Spanish). The model also has attracted some following in more distant parts of the world—in Africa, Australia,
South America, India and the Far East, for example—as we know
either from sales of *The Elements of Nursing* or from direct contact.
The recent inclusion of the Roper-Logan-Tierney model in two
American texts (Hinton-Walker & Neuman 1997, Marriner Tomey
& Alligood 1998) reflects recognition now in North America
of this British nursing model and, more generally, a recognition
there of the growing European contribution to theoretical
nursing.

However, while these are indicators of widespread interest in
the Roper-Logan-Tierney model, the *impact* of any particular
nursing model is difficult to gauge. Surveys conducted in North
America (e.g. Hall 1979, Jacobson 1987) have found familiarity
with the well-established conceptual frameworks, but evidence of
direct use of a model in practice is less easy to obtain. In the UK,
Jukes (1988) reportedly found that nursing models were seen
mostly as 'a classroom matter' although, by some of those sur-
veyed, they were also regarded as providing frameworks for
patient assessment, and the Roper-Logan-Tierney model was the
most favoured in the areas investigated.

The Roper-Logan-Tierney model certainly has been widely
taught in British colleges of nursing over the years and, where
a model has been used in practice, it has been one of the most
popular in the UK. Of course, how *well* it is used cannot be

gauged and it has to be said that claimed 'use' of our model sometimes has amounted to little more than adoption of its ALs terminology in nursing documentation without obvious use of the other concepts in the model. However, some evidence of well-considered use of the model in practice and in education is to be found in the nursing literature, and over the years we have come across at least 40 articles that report use of our model. A comprehensive, systematic search of the literature is difficult, however, because the model is seldom named in titles or key-words, and sometimes it is not referenced directly in an article even although the content, whether implicitly or explicitly, does in fact draw on the Roper-Logan-Tierney list of ALs or the model as a whole.

Contribution of the model

The contribution which the Roper-Logan-Tierney model has made to the theory or practice of nursing is impossible to assess objectively. Before examining the expressed views of others, we offer our own appraisal. In particular, we want to highlight some aspects of the model's conceptualization of nursing that, arguably, were innovative (even if not unique) at the time of its first publication and which we consider still have relevance now and for the future.

Reframing nursing's relationship with medicine

We believe that the model was innovative, at least in the British context, in providing a way of conceptualizing nursing in which the *independent* (i.e. nurse-initiated) rather than the *dependent* (i.e. medically delegated) aspects of practice were given pre-eminence. Through its focus on ALs and the individuality of patients/clients, the model did provide a way of loosening nurs-ing from its long-standing adherence to the medical (i.e. disease-focused) model that has dominated twentieth century healthcare in the Western world. But, at the same time, we emphasized the close relationship between the ALs and the body systems in order to provide a clear bridge between the doctor's concern with a patient's disease condition and a nurse's concern with that patient's wider needs arising from the effect of the disease on the individual's ALs. To have detached nursing from medicine in a more radical way would have been, we believe, both unacceptable and inappropriate.

But not everyone agrees with that. Biley (1992) has argued that our model represents little more than a change of labels: for example, a relabelling of the respiratory system to the AL of breathing. In defence of such criticisms, Parker (1997) suggested that the Roper-Logan-Tierney model has been berated excessively as a 'medically oriented, materialistic, reductionist approach' and cautioned that 'we too easily discard something which is easy to comprehend, straightforward and actually works in conjunction with medical practice'. The fact that our model is seen, at least by some, as a framework that can coexist with the medical model may yet prove to be one of its particular strengths as the call increases for doctors and nurses, and indeed all members of the healthcare team, to work more closely together in the day-to-day care of patients, families and communities.

Shifting the emphasis from ill-health to health

Similarly we would claim that our model's focus on *Activities of Living* also provided a way of shifting the emphasis in nursing from ill-health to health. Although a 'health orientation' was beginnning to gain ground, its operationalization in everyday nursing practice was very limited at the time we began work on our model. It was, after all, not until the late 1970s that the World Health Organization began to promote the concept of Primary Health Care (WHO / UNICEF 1978). And now, in the 1990s, *health targets* are being promoted by governments across the world in recognition that the major gains from healthcare investment will result not from medical advances, but from changes in personal lifestyle. A model for nursing centred on the concept of ALs could not be more relevant in this context. It fits well with the concept of 'health-promoting nursing practice' and we do not accept, on grounds of its excessive polarization, the argument put forward by Lindsey & Hartrick (1996) that an emphasis on health promotion is incompatible with paradigms (such as our model) that embrace the nursing process. We believe that our model is entirely congruent with the ever-increasing emphasis on healthy lifestyle and healthy public policy, and these trends, now gaining momentum, are unlikely to be reversed.

Complexity of nursing

Our model also contributed, and still provides, through the concept of *factors influencing the ALs*, a way of appreciating the breadth and complexity of the individuality of patients, families and communities. Health and illness are products of a complex array, and interaction of, internal and external factors. The inclusion of *biological* and *psychological* factors in the model was nothing novel in the 1970s and the relevance of *sociocultural* factors was gaining acceptance in nursing. Attention to *environmental* factors, however, was not well developed and, without doubt, the inclusion of *politicoeconomic* factors in our model was novel at the time, although now is an integral aspect of healthcare systems all over the world.

Individualizing nursing

Perhaps the most immediate contribution of our model was in terms of the framework it offered for operationalizing the nursing process. Ironically, the model's explicit adoption of the nursing process may well be a reason now for its rejection, at least in those circles where disparagement of the nursing process has become the new dogma (Varcoe 1996). The values that underpin the model's conceptualization of individualized nursing, however, are essentially the same as the ideas that came to be described as the 'New Nursing' (Salvage 1990) and, indeed, there is nothing in the model that is essentially incompatible with the more recent interests that have developed in nursing around the idea of 'caring' and the ideals of empowerment.

Making nursing theory accessible

Finally, we suggest that the Roper-Logan-Tierney model has made—and continues to make—a positive contribution to nursing by presenting 'nursing theory' in a form that is accessible and acceptable to practising nurses. Clarity of language surrounding a model has been said to reflect clarity of thinking (Cormack & Reynolds 1992). With regard to our model, Girot (1990) considers that its apparent simplicity has encouraged recognition of common ground in communication between theorists and practitioners. The Roper-Logan-Tierney model appears to reflect what

Meleis (1997) refers to as 'a coherent representation of the dailiness of nurses' work'. Newton (1992) concludes her assessment of
our model by commending its grounding in reality:

The Roper-Logan-Tierney model is based on ideas derived from
practice and may be seen to be useful in practice—for real nurses,
nursing real people.

Although a 'gap' between theory and practice in nursing may
be inevitable, and even desirable (Rafferty et al 1996), theory that
has no semblance of reality and is mystified by jargon is unlikely
to impinge on nurses in practice. Timpson (1996) believes that
the common perception of nurse theorists as removed from
the realities of practice is a major reason, compounded by 'rhetor-
ical élitism', for rejection of nursing theory by practising nurses. In
contrast, the realism and accessibility of the Roper-Logan–Tierney
model have been reasons for its impact and its survival.

Criticisms of the model

We move on now to look in greater detail at what others have had
to say about our model. In general, the view of the Roper-Logan-
Tierney model appears to be positively balanced, at least on the
basis of available evidence. Outright condemnation of the model
has been rare, at least in published form. One of the earliest published 'attacks' on our model came from a British consultant
physician (Mitchell 1984; see also Tierney 1984), although, in fact,
it seemed that the overly complicated documentation being used
in his ward in connection with the model was really his major
concern. Indeed, it was really the nursing process—rather than
our model—that lay at the root of his criticisms.

In contrast, one of the most vocal critics of our model from
within *nursing* circles in the UK has berated the oversimplicity,
rather than complexity, of the model (Walsh 1991). Its apparent
lack of novelty has also been criticized: as mentioned already,
Biley (1992) saw no fresh conceptualization in our model and
Lister (1991) expressed a similar viewpoint in suggesting that our
model allows nurses to preserve the status quo; does not provide
'a new perspective on nursing activity'; and does not appear to
'challenge entrenched viewpoints'. We must leave readers to
decide for themselves.

Nurses' views

Aside from views on the model that can be found in the published literature, other nurses have offered their opinions on the model in person, either in conversation at conferences or in correspondence. Initially, most of the concerns and criticisms put to us were on points of detail and from nurses who were trying to 'implement' the model in practice, for example questions such as 'Which AL does bleeding fit into?', 'Where does pain fit in the model?'. Some of the broader issues raised with us have portrayed more general concerns, for example that the model is 'too hospital orientated' (in response, we have made more explicit references to the community context in each new edition of *The Elements of Nursing*) or that it is 'too problem orientated' (although this, we contend, is not a valid criticism if our conceptualization of problems in the model as *potential* as well as *actual* is fully exploited). Indeed, these concerns tend to disappear when the model is actually tried out; for example, Page (1995) concludes that the criticism of our model as narrowly concerned with 'the adult hospital setting' is not borne out when it is applied in the community setting, and case studies of patients being nursed at home, within the framework of the model, are presented by way of illustration.

Fraser's critique

The single most comprehensive critique of the Roper-Logan-Tierney model which has been presented to date is to be found in Fraser's book entitled *Using Conceptual Nursing in Practice* (Fraser 1990, 1996). It should be noted, however, that the first edition of Fraser's book concentrates on the *first* edition of our model (1980), even though the second edition of *The Elements of Nursing* (1985) was available at the time. Our ongoing refinement of the model is not acknowledged and indeed there is little evidence in Fraser's later edition (1996) of any serious reflection or reconsideration of her original critique of our model.

One of Fraser's points of criticism is one that has been frequently levelled at our model: namely, that it is overly physically—and physiologically—orientated. This point has been made, or alluded to, by a number of writers (Aggleton & Chalmers 1986, Lister 1987, Minschull et al 1986, Walsh 1989). That common criticism, however, is openly rejected by Newton (1992) who, having written a book on *The Roper-Logan-Tierney Model in Action*, considers that the repeated emphasis in our model on all dimensions of the ALs (i.e. through the concept of *factors influencing the ALs*) does allow due emphasis to be placed on psychosocial dimensions of patients' problems and need not result in a narrowly 'physical' perception of patients' needs and nursing interventions. Similarly, Parker (1997) points out that, in spite of as much emphasis in the model on the 'psychosocial' as on the 'physical' factors, the former have simply not been exploited in systems of patient assessment and care planning that purport to be based on the Roper-Logan-Tierney model. Indeed, there is evidence suggesting that, when attempting to base their assessment system on a nursing model, the features of that model are not exploited: in other words, this is a problem not specific to *our* model, but to models in general. Griffiths (1998) investigated how nurses in two wards in a hospital in Wales (UK) were documenting patients' problems, one ward using the Roper-Logan-Tierney model and the other using Orem's 'self-care' model (Orem 1980). The study concluded that 'neither ward effectively applied the concepts of their espoused nursing model to their practice', both tending to express patients' problems in terms of conventional medical terminology.

Fraser's analysis of our model then proceeds by summarizing published accounts of its reported use, highlighting in turn those reports that focus on the steps of assessment, identification of problems, planning/implementation and evaluation. Fraser reports having found only one study (Allan 1987) that attempted to *test* an aspect of our model, and she places much emphasis on this finding as reflected in the overall conclusion of her assessment of the Roper-Logan-Tierney model:

Many . . . studies have shown the use of the model in practice, but none have taken a systematic approach to data collection and therefore cannot be said to be testing the model in practice. However, that the model has been so widely used in so many different practice areas shows its acceptability to nurses in Great Britain.

Declining interest in the model?

In the later edition of her book, however, Fraser (1996) suggests that there is evidence of 'the decline of this model's popularity'.

She makes this assertion on the basis of having found no new studies of our model since 1990 except for one unfavourable comparison against American frameworks (Parr 1993). In fact, Fraser had missed a number of other post-1990 publications on the model and, since the second edition of her book (Fraser 1996), further papers on the Roper-Logan-Tierney model have appeared in the nursing press. Examples include:

- Newton's (1992) book on the Roper-Logan-Tierney model 'in action', as mentioned already
- McCaugherty's (1992) report of use of the model as the basis of an educational and research tool
- Rowe's (1995) case study of a patient who had suffered a myocardial infarction, showing the value found in our model in terms of encouraging exploration of the uniqueness of each patient and the unique needs of the family members
- Bellman's (1996) account of an action research study that used the model to promote reflective practice
- Davis's (1997) adaptation of the model, centred around the AL of mobilizing, for use in orthopaedic nursing
- Ramsden's (1997) description of finding the model helpful in reflecting on her involvement in the care of a dying patient in the setting of a nursing home
- Pullen's (1998) report of having found the model to be helpful as a framework for the care of patients with a stoma, highlighting the value of AL-driven assessment in assisting patients to 'acquire, maintain or restore maximum independence'
- Jones' (1998) discussion of the needs of a patient undergoing pharyngeal surgery through a detailed focus on the ALs of eating and drinking and communicating.

These are just a selection of publications that, drawing on the Roper-Logan-Tierney model, have been published since Fraser's (1996) assertion of declining interest in the model. It is, of course, impossible to gauge whether or not the level of interest is rising or falling, but the fact that the model continues to be referenced in the literature, including reports of its use in practice, suggests that interest in it has not declined or, at least, certainly has not dried up completely.

In most of the published reports, the comments about the model tend to be more positive than negative. There are, of course, some exceptions to this. Scott (1997), for example, reports that use of the Roper-Logan-Tierney model in a project designed to improve care plans in a stroke rehabilitation unit failed to 'reflect the philosophy of rehabilitation' and failed to 'increase patients' independence'. Whether these were failures of the model, or a failure to exploit the model, cannot be properly judged. But, in any case, attributing patient outcomes to use of the model assumes that a nursing model can be empirically *tested*.

Concern about lack of testing

Fraser's main criticism of our model, then, is that it has not been *tested* and, on this basis, she concludes that 'the effectiveness of nursing care using the Roper-Logan-Tierney model is still speculative'. Admittedly, one of the main intentions of Fraser's book was to uncover the knowledge that has been accumulated from *research* about the use of nursing models in practice. Rightly, Fraser notes that the Roper-Logan-Tierney model has not generated research, at least not to the same extent as some of the other (American) models, such as those of Roy, Orem, Johnson and Rogers, which are also put under scrutiny in Fraser's book. However, given that Fraser defines a model at the outset of her book as 'a set of concepts that *have not yet been tested out* in practice' (italics added), it does seem somewhat contradictory that her conclusions about the Roper-Logan-Tierney model appear to be driven by concern that the model has not been adequately tested. This raises an interesting general question about models of nursing: can and should they be tested?

The 'testing' of models

For the Roper-Logan-Tierney model, and for all conceptual models of nursing, the question of whether they should (and can) be tested has become crucial to the debate about whether or not models should be accorded a continuing place in nursing theory. Definition of what a 'model' is and views about how 'theory' is developed are fundamental to discussion of this question.

As defined by Fawcett (1984), a conceptual model is not a theory and, therefore—at least in its entirety—a model cannot be empirically tested as a whole. Evaluation of a conceptual model can be accomplished, in Fawcett's view, only by examining its content in terms of 'explication of origins, comprehensiveness of focus and content, logical congruence, credibility and contribution to nursing knowledge' (Fawcett 1995). Fawcett insists that the 'goodness' of a model must be judged primarily in terms of the notion of 'credibility', whereas the 'goodness' of a theory hinges on the notion of empirical adequacy (Fawcett & Downs 1986).

Assessing credibility

What Fawcett means by the notion of 'credibility' is explained further by Kahn & Fawcett (1995), in a paper primarily intended as an exposé of flaws in Draper's (1993) critique of Fawcett's (1992) paper on conceptual models. Kahn & Fawcett assert that the credibility of a conceptual model requires evidence of:

- social utility (i.e. its 'understandability' and potential for utility)
- social congruence (i.e. its fit with social and professional expectations)
- social significance (i.e. its value, particularly for patients).

With regard to the Roper-Logan-Tierney model, there does appear to be evidence of its social utility and social congruence: these ideas are embodied in Fraser's (1990) overall evaluation of our model in terms of its 'acceptability' to nurses. And, on the basis of its widespread use, the Roper-Logan-Tierney model also appears to fulfil the criteria of the third dimension of credibility—social significance—although, admittedly, this has not been subjected to analysis by the systematic method that Kahn & Fawcett (1995) set out in the form of a six-step approach based on Silva (1986). Description of that approach, however, is rather difficult to follow and, indeed, Fawcett's interest in Silva's work is somewhat perplexing. While Fawcett is so disciplined in her use of terminology and fiercely opposes the idea of the empirical testing of models, Silva (1986) uses the terms 'model' and 'theory' somewhat loosely, and her driving concern is about the lack of 'empirical validation of the models'. Admittedly, Silva acknowledges the complex nature of theory-testing research and she recognizes that 'dozens of hypotheses' can be deduced from any single model. Despite this, Silva seems adamant that the 'validity' of models must be tested through empirical research.

In contrast, Fawcett rejects 'a verificationist methodology' (Kahn & Fawcett 1995). If Fawcett's stance is accepted, then calls for conceptual models to be 'tested' are misguided and the proposition that models should not be presented as 'untested theory' (e.g. Cormack & Reynolds 1992) is discredited, despite being a popular call in some circles. But readers must make up their own minds about whether a nursing model should (and can be) 'tested'. If, however, Fawcett's arguments are accepted, then there is no case for the *testing* of models and, therefore, no grounds for the dismissal of the Roper-Logan-Tierney model on grounds that it has not been empirically tested.

Research and critique of models

Dismissal of the call for the 'testing' of a model as an entity is not, of course, a rejection of the need to conduct research that can exploit the theory-generating capacity of nursing models, nor is it a rejection of the need for ongoing critique. Fawcett herself states clearly that nursing models should not be regarded as 'ideologies that must not be questioned or criticized' (Fawcett 1992). It is mandatory, she states, that their credibility in the 'real world' of clinical practice should be questioned closely and, as a result, there should be 'subsequent refinement or elimination of the model'.

This requirement applies to the Roper-Logan-Tierney model as it does to all nursing models and, indeed, we have stated repeatedly that our model is not set in marble and should be discarded when it is no longer considered to be meaningful for nursing. It has been our position, however, to leave *others* to engage in systematic critique and objective research which relates to our model rather than to engage in that ourselves. Indeed, Thorne et al (1998) direct criticism at those 'model builders' who themselves have initiated research that promotes their own particular framework and they are sceptical about 'the efforts of model builders to build communities of scholars towards the purpose of developing and furthering particular models'. Thorne et al suggest that this has inhibited the development of a critical attitude towards nursing models and contend that, although debate and discourse within a discipline can be healthy and productive, 'the model debate was rarely elevated to that level'.

We hope that the assessment of the Roper-Logan-Tierney model presented in this chapter, drawing not only on our own reflections on the model but also on the criticisms and views of others that have been published over time, will serve to encourage ongoing and critical debate.

Looking to the future

It is interesting to ponder whether or not nursing models will continue to play an ongoing role in the future development of nursing knowledge. In her treatise on nursing knowledge for the twenty-first century, Reed (1995) strongly rejects the idea that nursing has matured beyond needing conceptual models for knowledge development and for practice. She recognizes that, from a post-modernist stance, the 'grand' or 'high' theories of the modernists are viewed as oppressive fabrications rather than meaningful representations of reality. For post-modernists, Reed observes, problems are not 'solved' but are 'deconstructed' and she attributes their recoil from nursing models as symptomatic of their 'disinterest in grappling with the wholes that grand-level theories address'.

But, arguably, with ever-increasing scrutiny of nursing's contribution in today's fast-changing world of health care, the profession is surely as much—if not more—in need of a sense of clarity about its core values and central concepts as it was when the early nurse theorists began this task of 'grappling with the whole' by trying to answer the age-old question: 'What is nursing?'.

The question 'What is nursing?' is a *conceptual* question and a nursing model is a way of *conceptualizing* the domain of nursing. Many of the original nursing models still survive and are still taught to nursing students and used by practising nurses and nurse scholars. It will be interesting to see whether the original American models of the mid-twentieth century, and our own model of nursing, will continue to attract interest in future years; or whether newer models will take their place; or whether models will go out of fashion altogether, eventually to be consigned to the history books as a 'phase' of late twentieth century nursing, albeit with acknowledgement that they provided a 'useful step' in the early stages of knowledge development of nursing.

If the notion of nursing models does survive over time, there will continue to be argument about whether it is helpful—or confusing—for the profession to have a variety of nursing models in play—what Fawcett (1993) calls a 'plethora of paradigms'. Reed

(1995) is ambivalent on this issue. She questions whether co-herence in nursing science is not being sacrificed for diversity and, indeed, whether diversity best serves the well-being of patients. However, on the question of whether nursing needs 'high level' conceptualization, Reed has no doubts at all. She con-tends that the articulation of disciplinary perspectives and under-lying assumptions is a necessary mechanism for knowledge development in nursing; all disciplines, she argues, require study of the 'particulars' to be grounded in the 'universals'. 'Grand' theory need not hamper the vital task of research in seeking to generate 'low' and 'middle-range' theories for nursing but, with-out it, there will be no sense of place for that new knowledge and no clarity of overall direction for the development of the discipline.

Reed's vision for the twenty-first century is one in which mod-ernist and post-modernist thinking coexist in nursing science (what she calls the 'neo-modernist era') and, in that respect, her ideas reflect the call that Meleis has been putting out over recent years for nursing scholarship to advance beyond dualism and adversarial argument (Meleis & Trangenstein 1994). In Reed's vision for the future, both empirical and non-empirical (concep-tual) thinking are accorded a place, and different forms of know-ledge are not ordered hierarchically. As she observes, approaches to linking the 'empirical' and the 'theoretical' have changed over the history of nursing science, and will continue to do so. What is Reed's final word on nursing models? 'Nursing models are more than a modernist artefact', she asserts: 'they are archetypes of nursing practice'. But, at the same time, she cautions that they must be seen as 'open and alterable'. As systems of knowledge, Reed argues, nursing models must continue to evolve 'lest they move from being extant to becoming extinct'.

We hope that *our* nursing model will continue to evolve through its use and adaptation in the future. Although this mono-graph presents our final account of the Roper-Logan-Tierney model, it need not be the final version.

REFERENCES

Aggleton P, Chalmers H 1986, 2000 Nursing models and the nursing process, 1st & 2nd edn. Macmillan Educational, Basingstoke, UK
Allan S 1987 Arms extended. Nursing Times 83(43):44–45

Bellman L M 1996 Changing practice through reflection on the Roper, Logan and Tierney model: the enhancement approach to action research. Journal of Advanced Nursing 24:129–138

Biley F 1992 Nursing models redundant in practice. British Journal of Nursing 1(5):219

Cash K 1990 Nursing models and the idea of nursing. International Journal of Nursing Studies 27(3):249–256

Chalmers H, Kershaw B, Melia K, Kendrich M 1990 Clinical nursing debates. Nursing Standard 5(11):34–40

Cormack D F S, Reynolds W 1992 Criteria for evaluating the clinical and practical utility of models used by nurses. Journal of Advanced Nursing 17:1472–1478

Davis P 1997 Using models and theories in orthopaedic nursing. Journal of Orthopaedic Nursing 1:41–47

Draper P 1990 The development of theory in British nursing: current position and future prospects. Journal of Advanced Nursing 15:12–15

Draper P 1993 A critique of Fawcett's 'Conceptual models and nursing practice: the reciprocal relationship. Journal of Advanced Nursing 18:558–564

Fawcett J 1984, 1989, 1995 Analysis and evaluation of conceptual models for nursing, 1st, 2nd & 3rd edn. H A Davis, Philadelphia

Fawcett J 1992 Conceptual models and nursing practice: the reciprocal relationship. Journal of Advanced Nursing 17:224–228

Fawcett J 1993 From a plethora of paradigms to parsimony in worldviews. Nursing Science Quarterly 6:56–58

Fawcett J, Downs F S 1986 The relationship of theory and research. Appleton-Century-Crofts, Norwalk, Connecticut

Fraser M 1990,1996 Using conceptual nursing in practice: a research-based approach, 1st & 2nd edn. Harper & Row, London

Girot E 1990 Discussing nursing theory. Senior Nurse 10(6):16–19

Griffiths P 1998 An investigation into the description of patients' problems by nurses using two different needs-based nursing models. Journal of Advanced Nursing 28(5):969–977

Hall K V 1979 Current trends in the use of conceptual frameworks in nursing education. Journal of Nurse Education 18(4):26–29

Henderson V 1960 Basic principles of nursing care. International Council of Nurses, Geneva

Hinton-Walker P, Neuman B 1997 Blueprint for use of nursing models. NLN Press, New York

Jacobson S 1987 Studying and using conceptual models of nursing. Image 19(2): 78–83

Jones E 1998 Surgical excision of a pharyngeal pouch. Professional Nurse 13(6):378–381

Jukes M 1988 Nursing model or psychological assessment? Senior Nurse 8(11):8–10

Kahn S, Fawcett J 1995 Continuing the dialogue: a response to Draper's critique of Fawcett's 'Conceptual models and nursing practice: the reciprocal relationship'. Journal of Advanced Nursing 22:188–192

Kenny T 1993 Nursing models fail in practice. British Journal of Nursing 2:133–136

Kershaw B, Salvage J (eds) 1986 Models for nursing. John Wiley, Chichester, UK

Lindsey E, Hartrick G 1996 Health-promoting nursing practice: the demise of the nursing process? Journal of Advanced Nursing 23:106–112

Lister P E 1987 The misunderstood model. Nursing Times 83(41):40–42

Lister P E 1991 Approaching models of nursing from a postmodernist perspective. Journal of Advanced Nursing 16:206–212

Luker K 1988 Do models work? Nursing Times 88(5):27–29

Marriner Tomey A, Alligood MR 1998 Nurse theorists and their work, 4th edn. Mosby, St Louis

McCaugherty D 1992 The Roper nursing model as an educational and research tool. British Journal of Nursing 1(9):455–459

Meleis A I 1985, 1991, 1997 Theoretical nursing: development and progress, Ist, 2nd & 3rd edn. J B Lippincott, Philadelphia

Meleis A I, Trangenstein PA 1994 Facilitating transitions: redefinition of the nursing mission. Nursing Outlook 42:255–259

Minschull J, Rose K, Turner J 1986 The human needs model of nursing. Journal of Advanced Nursing 11:643–649

Mitchell J R A 1984 Is nursing any business of doctors? A simple guide to the 'nursing process'. British Medical Journal 288:216–219

Newton C 1992 The Roper-Logan-Tierney model in action. Macmillan, Hampshire

Nursing Development Conference Group 1973 Concept formalization in nursing: process and product. Little, Brown, New York

Orem D 1971 Nursing: concepts of practice. McGraw-Hill, New York

Orem D 1980 Nursing: concepts of practice, 2nd edn. McGraw-Hill, New York

Page M 1995 Tailoring nursing models to clients' needs: using the Roper-Logan-Tierney model after discharge. Professional Nurse 10(5):284–288

Parker D 1997 Nursing art and science: literature and debate. In: Marks-Maran D, Rose P (eds) Reconstructing nursing: beyond art and science. Baillière Tindall, London, ch 1, p 3

Parr M S 1993 The Newman Health Care Systems Model: an evaluation. British Journal of Theatre Nursing 3(8):20–27

Pearson A, Vaughan B 1986, 1996 The activities of living model for nursing. In: Pearson A, Vaughan B (eds) Nursing models for practice, 1st & 2nd edn. Heinemann, London

Pullen M 1998 Support role. Nursing Times 94(47):57

Rafferty A M, Allcock N, Lathlean J 1996 The theory/practice 'gap': taking issue with the issue. Journal of Advanced Nursing 23:685–691

Ramsden J 1997 Objective analysis of a critical incident. Nursing Times 93(34):43–45

Reed P G 1995 A treatise on nursing knowledge development in the 21st century: beyond postmodernism. Advances in Nursing Science 17(3):70–84

Reilly D 1975 Why a conceptual framework? Nursing Outlook 23:566–569

Riehl J, Roy C 1980 Conceptual models for nursing practice. Appleton-Century-Crofts, New York

Rogers M 1970 An introduction to the theoretical basis of nursing. F A Davis, Philadelphia

Roper N 1976a Clinical experience in nurse education. Churchill Livingstone, Edinburgh

Roper N 1976b A model for nursing and nursology. Journal of Advanced Nursing 1(3):219–227

Roper N 1979 Nursing based on a model of living. In: Colledge M, Jones D (eds) Readings in Nursing. Churchill Livingstone, Edinburgh, ch 6

Roper N, Logan W, Tierney A 1980, 1985, 1990, 1996 The elements of nursing: a model for nursing based on a model of living, 1st, 2nd, 3rd & 4th edn. Churchill Livingstone, Edinburgh

Roper N, Logan W, Tierney A 1981 Learning to use the process of nursing. Churchill Livingstone, Edinburgh

Roper N, Logan W, Tierney A (eds) 1983a Using a model for nursing. Churchill Livingstone, Edinburgh

Roper N, Logan W, Tierney A 1983b A model for nursing. Nursing Times 9(9):24–27

Roper N, Logan W, Tierney A 1983c (1) A nursing model, (2) Is there a danger of 'processing' patients?, (3) Problems or needs?, (4) Identifying the goals, (5) Endless paperwork?, (6) Unity—with diversity. Nursing Mirror 156(21):17–19; 156(22):32–33; 156(23):43–44; 156(24):22–23; 156(25):34–35; 156(26):35

Roper N, Logan W, Tierney A 1986 Nursing models: a process of construction and refinement. In: Salvage J, Kershaw B (eds) Models for nursing. John Wiley, Chichester, UK, p 27

Roper N, Logan W, Tierney A 1997 The Roper-Logan-Tierney model. In: Hinton-Walker P, Neuman B (eds) Blueprint for use of nursing models. NLN Press, New York, p 289

Rowe K 1995 Nursing a person who had suffered a myocardial infarction. British Journal of Nursing 4(3):148–154

Roy C 1970 Adaptation: a conceptual framework for nursing. Nursing Outlook 18(3):42–45

Salvage J 1990 The theory and practice of the 'new nursing'. Nursing Times 86(4):42–45

Silva M C 1986 Research testing nursing theory: state of the art. Advances in Nursing Science 9(1):1–11

Scott E 1997 Multidisciplinary collaborative care planning. Nursing Standard 12(1):39–42

Thorne S, Canam C, Dahinten S, Hall W, Henderson A, Reimer Kirkham S 1998 Nursing's metaparadigm concepts: disimpacting the debate. Journal of Advanced Nursing 27:1257–1268

Tierney A J 1984 A response to Professor Mitchell's 'Simple guide to the nursing process'. British Medical Journal 288:835–838

Timpson J 1996 Nursing theory: everything the artist spits is art. Journal of Advanced Nursing 23:1030–1036

Varcoe C 1996 Disparagement of the nursing process: the new dogma? Journal of Advanced Nursing 23:120–125

Walsh M 1989 Model example. Nursing Standard 3:23–25

Walsh M 1991 Models in clinical nursing: the way forward. Baillière Tindall, London

WHO/UNICEF 1978 Primary health care. World Health Organization, Geneva

Appendix 1

ALTERATIONS IN THE DIAGRAMMATIC REPRESENTATION OF THE MODELS FROM 1976 TO 1996

The original Roper models, 1976

Figures A1. 1a and b show the diagrams of the models produced by Roper (1976) in *Clinical Experience in Nurse Education*. This was a monograph based on her Master of Science thesis.

The Elements of Nursing, 1980 (first edition)

Roper, Logan and Tierney collaborated to develop the original Roper models, and published the results of their thinking and discussions in *The Elements of Nursing* in 1980. As mentioned earlier, this textbook was intended, essentially, for beginning students to introduce them to a way of 'thinking' about nursing—a theoretical base for nursing practice. The diagrams in Figures A1.2a and b are a reflection of the text and differed from the original Roper models in the following ways:

- The term 'Activities of Daily Living' (ADLs) was replaced by 'Activities of Living' (ALs) in recognition of the fact that all of them are not necessarily 'daily'.
- The ADLs of talking, seeing, hearing and socializing were combined to be the AL of communicating, which was considered to encompass a wider range of activities including, for example, 'listening' and 'body language'.
- The ADL of feeding was changed to the AL of eating and drinking; this made more explicit the fact that fluid intake was a crucial aspect of body physiology.
- The ADL of working and the ADL of playing were combined to be the AL of working and playing.

- The ADL of cleansing and the ADL of dressing became the AL of personal cleansing and dressing.
- The ADL of relaxing and the ADL of sleeping became the AL of sleeping.
- Four new ALs were added:
  — maintaining a safe environment
  — controlling body temperature
  — expressing sexuality
  — dying.

At the time of our writing in the late 1970s, it was only beginning to be fashionable to consider *environmental* issues.

In 1980, when the first edition of *The Elements of Nursing* was published, the inclusion of the AL of *expressing sexuality* was greeted with considerable surprise. Obviously, from the vantage point of the year 2000, with all the media coverage about sex and sexuality, such a reaction seems bizarre.

Strange as it may seem in 2000, specific discussions about *dying* and death were only beginning to appear in the national basic curriculum in the 1980s, so the inclusion of the AL of dying was an innovation (such discussions had been included in the degree programme for nursing at the University of Edinburgh in the 1960s when Logan was the course organizer).

- The currently accepted (1980) nomenclature of the nursing process was used (see Fig. A1.2b).

During the 1970s, the American literature about the nursing process was gaining recognition in the UK. Although the same ideas were conveyed in the Roper model of 1976, the actual words 'assessing', planning', 'implementing' and 'evaluating' were used in the first publication about the Roper-Logan-Tierney models (Fig. A1.2b).

The Elements of Nursing, 1985 (second edition)

Throughout their work, Roper, Logan and Tierney have welcomed written and verbal comments from users and critics of their models, and have used this information to clarify their subsequent writing and the accompanying diagrammatic representations of their thinking. Changes made in the second edition of *The Elements of Nursing* are shown in Figures A1.3a and b.

- The diagrams were redesigned.

- The dependence/independence continuum was depicted as a continuum alongside each AL in order to make it visually clearer that the individual's capacity for dependence or independence may not be the same for all 12 ALs.
- A separate concept entitled 'Factors influencing Activities of Living' was added to the diagrams in an attempt to emphasize visually that each factor (physical, psychological, sociocultural, environmental, politicoeconomic) could be related to each of the 12 ALs. This was intended to give ample scope for using accepted concepts from disciplines related to nursing—'shared knowledge' according to Fawcett (1984, 1995)—and applying them in nursing practice. During the late 1970s, in the national basic nursing curriculum, aspects of psychology and sociology were only beginning to be introduced (they had been included as separate disciplines for study in the degree programme for nursing at the University of Edinburgh in the 1960s, and relevant content was applied to nursing theory and practice).
- A separate concept was added: individuality in living.

  The four other concepts of the model of living—the 12 ALs, the lifespan, the dependence/independence continuum, the factors influencing the ALs—were combined to indicate the unique mix that contributes to the fifth concept of individuality of living.
- A different name was given to the process of nursing, namely, 'individualizing nursing'.

  The four other concepts of the model of nursing—the 12 ALs, the lifespan, the dependence/independence continuum, the factors influencing the ALs—were combined to indicate the fifth concept of 'individualizing nursing', accomplished by using the method of logical thinking known as the nursing process. It is not possible to individualize nursing unless one takes into account the person's individuality in living.

The Elements of Nursing, 1990 (third edition)

The diagrams of the models in the third edition, seen in Figures A1.4a and b were similar to Figures A1.3a and b in the second edition, but were redesigned to look less 'cluttered'.

The Elements of Nursing, 1996 (fourth edition)

The diagrams of the models in the fourth edition were unchanged except for one word in the factors: 'biological' replaced 'physical', as seen in Figures A1.5a and b.

(a)

ACTIVITIES Performed by most people	Conception ——————— Lifetime span ——————— Death
	Dependent ···········Continuum··········· Independent circumstances

	Breathing
ACTIVITIES	Feeding
OF	Eliminating
DAILY	Personal cleansing
LIVING	Dressing
(ADL)	Mobilizing
	*Talking
	Seeing
	Hearing
	Socializing
	Working
	Playing
	Relaxing
	Sleeping

*includes: eye talk, facial talk, touch talk

PREVENTING	COMFORTING	SEEKING
Performed by most people		

(b)

COMPONENTS Initiated by nurse for some patients Medically prescribed for other patients	Assessment	Objectives	Appropriate action	Evaluation

	Breathing
	Feeding
	Eliminating
	Personal cleansing
ADL	Dressing
	Mobilizing
	*Talking
	Seeing
	Hearing
	Socializing
	Working
	Playing
	Relaxing
	Sleeping

*includes: eye talk, facial talk, touch talk

PREVENTING	COMFORTING	MEDICALLY
Initiated by nurse		PRESCRIBED

Figure A1.1 (a) The model of living; (b) the model of nursing. From Roper N **1976** Clinical experience in nurse education. Churchill Livingstone, Edinburgh.

(a)

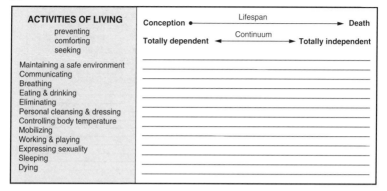

(b)

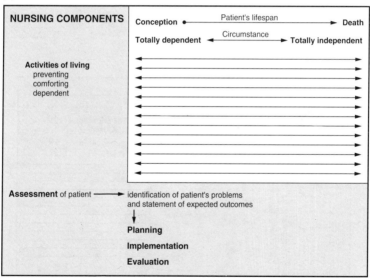

Figure A1.2   (a) The model of living; (b) the model of nursing. From Roper N, Logan W, Tierney A **1980** The elements of nursing. Churchill Livingstone, Edinburgh.

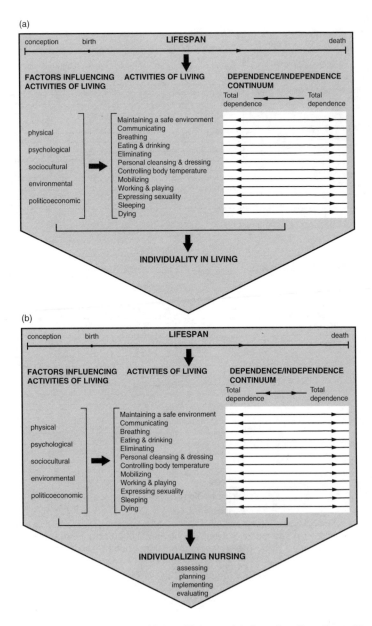

Figure A1.3   (a) The model of living; (b) the model of nursing. From Roper N, Logan W, Tierney A **1985** The elements of nursing, 2nd edn. Churchill Livingstone, Edinburgh.

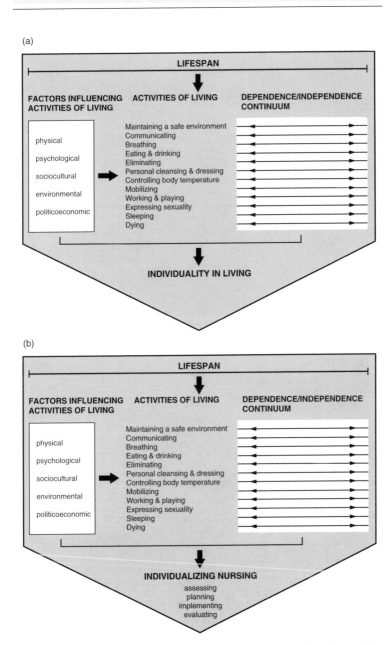

Figure A1.4   (a) The model of living; (b) the model of nursing. From Roper N, Logan W, Tierney A **1990** The elements of nursing, 3rd edn. Churchill Livingstone, Edinburgh.

(a)

(b)

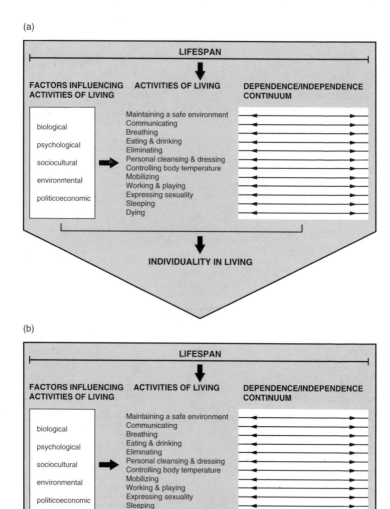

Figure A1.5 (a) The model of living; (b) the model of nursing. From Roper N, Logan W, Tierney A **1996** The elements of nursing, 4th edn. Churchill Livingstone, Edinburgh.

REFERENCES

Fawcett J 1984 Conceptual models of nursing. F A Davies, Philadelphia
Fawcett J 1995 Conceptual models of nursing, 3rd edn. F A Davies, Philadelphia
Roper N 1976 Clinical experience in nurse education. Churchill Livingstone,
     Edinburgh
Roper N, Logan W, Tierney A 1980, 1985, 1990, 1996 The elements of nursing,
     1st, 2nd, 3rd & 4th edn. Churchill Livingstone, Edinburgh

Appendix 2

EXAMPLE OF A PATIENT/CLIENT ASSESSMENT FORM AND NURSING PLAN

The type of information appropriate for patient assessment and for devising a nursing plan has already been discussed in general terms in Chapter 3. It cannot be emphasized too strongly that this pro forma (constructed initially for the third edition of The Elements of Nursing) is only a guideline. Many agencies have already devised a pro forma that suits their particular circumstances, and this example merely provides a guideline which could be helpful when using our model, whether in a community or a hospital setting.

It is worth making a few points about this particular document:

• Page one includes biographical and health data elicited at a first assessment. It does not usually change over a particular episode when nursing is required, but when an episode is prolonged in the community setting or a nursing home there may be some biographical change, for example the death of a spouse or close family member/significant other.

• Page two includes information about the person's Activities of Living (in so far as they reflect the person's stage on the lifespan and their dependence/independence status at the time of the assessment, and are influenced by biological, psychological, sociocultural, environmental and politicoeconomic factors). There is a reminder list on page two, but it may not be relevant to collect information about each of the 12 ALs. For example, nurses would have to use professional judgement regarding the appropriateness of collecting information about ALs when a client has only a brief contact with the health services such as attending a day surgery appointment (there is usually a pre-surgery interview), a clinic where investigations (e.g. gastroenterological procedures) are carried out on a day basis, or a short unscheduled visit as an outpatient to an accident and emergency unit.

The phrase 'usual routines' reflects the model's concept of individuality. The phrase 'what can/cannot be done independently' reflects the dependence/independence continuum; and 'previous coping mechanisms' reflects our concept of 'aided independence'. The person's actual problems are recorded on the right-hand side of page two, with potential problems designated by (p).

- Page three is for the nursing plan and forms the right side of a double fold so that problems identified at the initial assessment do not need to be recorded a second time. Goals are stated in outcome terms and a date for the evaluation of the selected nursing interventions can be entered. Once recorded, the nursing plan needs additional information only when:
  — a goal has been achieved
  — a nursing intervention has to be changed to achieve the goal already set
  — the goal has to be modified
  — the date of evaluation has to be changed
  — the person experiences further problems.

- Page four makes provision for interventions that may be medically prescribed or initiated by another member of the health team. Such information would not necessarily be documented in an AL format.

The 'other notes' section could be used for recording, for example clinic appointments or loans of equipment.

- Pages five and six make provision for more detailed items of information should a lengthy rehabilitation period be required in the community setting.

This pro forma was devised essentially for written records. The same type of information would be required on computerized records and/or as part of multiprofessional records, but the format would need to be suitably adapted.

Patient/Client Assessment Form: Biographical and health data		
Date of admission	Date of assessment	Nurse's signature
	Surname	Forenames

Male ☐   Age ☐
Female ☐

Date of birth _____
Single/Married/Widowed/Other

Prefers to be addressed as

Address of usual residence

Type of accommodation
(incl. mode of entry if relevant)

Family/Others at this residence

Next of kin/Other contact person   Name   Address

Relationship   Tel. no.

Significant others
(incl. relatives/dependants/
visitors/helpers/neighbours)

Support services

Occupation

Religion/beliefs and relevant practices

Recent significant life events/crises

Patient's/client's perception of current health status

Carers' perception of patient's/client's health status if appropriate

Reason for coming into contact with the health service

Medical information (e.g. diagnosis, past history, allergies)

GP Address Tel. no.

Plans for discharge

Page one Roper-Logan-Tierney © Harcourt Publishers Limited 2000

Figure A2.1   Model of nursing.

Patient/Client Assessment Form: Assessment of ALs

REMINDER OF CONCEPTS	**Activity of living AL**	Date Usual routines: what can/cannot be done independently previous coping mechanisms	Patient's problems: actual/potential (p)
The 12 ALs Maintaining a safe environment Communicating Breathing Eating & drinking Eliminating Personal cleansing & dressing Controlling body temperature Mobilizing Working & playing Expressing sexuality Sleeping Dying Lifespan Dep/indep Factors Biological Psychological Sociocultural Environmental Politicoeconomic			

Page two Roper-Logan-Tierney © Harcourt Publishers Limited 2000

Figure A2.2 Model of nursing.

Nursing Plan: Related to ALs

Goals	Nurse-initiated nursing interventions related to ALs	Evaluation

Page three Roper-Logan-Tierney © Harcourt Publishers Limited 2000

Figure A2.3 Model of nursing.

Nursing Plan: Derived from medical/other prescription

Nursing interventions derived from medical/other prescription	Goals	Evaluation

Other Notes

Page four Roper-Logan-Tierney © Harcourt Publishers Limited 2000

Figure A2.4 Model of nursing.

Medications Prescribed

Date	Prescription	Dose	Route	Frequency	Discontinued

Treatment Prescribed

Date	Prescription	Frequency	Response	Discontinued

Page five Roper-Logan-Tierney

Figure A2.5 Model of nursing.

Equipment on Loan

Date	Article	Source	Returned

Appointments

Date	Place	Reasons	Conveyance	Arranged

Supportive Services

Service	Date	Remarks	Discontinued
Social worker			
Meals on wheels			
Home help			
Palliative care			
Twillght/night nursing			
Physiotherapy			
Occupational therapy			
Speech therapy			
Chiropody			
Day hospital			
Voluntary services			
Other			

Figure A2.6 Model of nursing.

Appendix 3

ASSESSMENT FRAMEWORK

Assessing, as one aspect of the process of nursing, has been discussed on p. 130. In *The Elements of Nursing* (fourth edition), the assessment of each of the individual 12 Activities of Living was presented in detail to demonstrate that, once conversant with the concepts of the model of nursing, the nurse can assess the client's relevant ALs in relation to lifespan, dependence/independence status, and the five factors. Examples of an assessment framework from the fourth edition are given in this appendix for only three of the 12 ALs: eating and drinking (Box A3.1), communicating (Box A3.2) and mobilizing (Box A3.3). These outlines are merely aides-mémoire—indicative of the nurse's conceptual framework—and obviously would not be used in this format on a patient/client's record.

In essence, the questions the nurse would have in mind while assessing are:

- How does the individual usually deal with this AL?
- What factors influence the way the individual carries out this AL?
- What does the individual understand about this AL?
- What are the individual's attitudes to this AL?
- Has the individual any long-standing difficulties with this AL and how have they been coped with?
- What problems, if any, does the person have at present with this AL, or seem likely to develop?

Box A3.1 Assessing the individual in the AL of eating and drinking

Lifespan: effect on eating and drinking
- Nutrition in utero
- Breast/bottle-feeding and weaning in infancy
- Increasing skills in eating and drinking during childhood
- Healthy diet during adolescence and adulthood
- Reduced appetite/potential nutritional deficiency in old age

Dependence/independence in eating and drinking
- Special utensils
- Mechanical aids
- Kitchen gadgets
- Special transport for shopping

Factors influencing eating and drinking
- Biological
  - state of mouth and teeth
  - swallowing
  - intact digestive system
  - nutrition
  - physical ability for shopping/preparing food
  - physical ability for taking food and drink
  - appetite/thirst regulation
- Psychological
  - intellectual capacity to procure and prepare food and drink
  - knowledge about diet and health
  - weight control
  - distorted body image
  - alcohol dependence/abuse
  - food hygiene
  - disposal of food waste
  - attitude to eating and drinking
  - emotional status/mood
  - likes and dislikes
- Sociocultural
  - family traditions
  - cultural idiosyncrasies
  - religious commendations/restrictions
- Environmental
  - climate and geographical position
  - facilities for procuring/growing food
  - distance from home to shopping area
  - availability of transport
  - means of cooking
  - means of storage
  - vectors and food spoilage
- Politicoeconomic
  - malnutrition/finance
  - choice of food and drink
  - quantity and quality of food and drink
  - current national goals about healthy diet

Box A3.2   Assessing the individual in the AL of communicating

Lifespan: effect on communicating
- Fetal growth and movement/birth cry
- Infancy and childhood—increasing skills/forming relationships
- Adolescence   —extension of skills/relationships
- Adulthood   —variety in skills/relationships
- Old age   —gradual loss of activity/reduction in skills and relationships

Dependence/independence in communicating
- Unimpaired body structure and function
- Visual aids
- Hearing aids
- Speech aids
- Electronic aids

Factors influencing communicating
- Biological   —intact body structure and function
                      —speaking/voice pitch
                      —hearing
                      —seeing
                      —reading
                      —writing
                      —gesticulating
- Psychological   —intelligence/range of vocabulary/learning
                      —self-confidence
                      —self-worth, perception of self, and effect on perception of others
                      —body image
                      —prevailing mood
                      —information giving, teaching and counselling
                      —assertiveness
                      —human relationships
- Sociocultural   —indigenous language
                      —dialect/accent
                      —vocabulary
                      —ethnicity and discrimination
                      —personal appearance/dress
                      —patterns of touching
                      —eye contact/gesticulation
                      —attitudes, values and beliefs
                      —dyads and groups
- Environmental   —temperature/ventilation
                      —light
                      —noise
                      —type/size of room
                      —arrangement of furniture
- Politicoeconomic   —income
                      —occupation
                      —communication channels/mass media
                      —information technology
                      —legislation to protect data/individual

Box A3.3   Assessing the individual in the AL of mobilizing

Lifespan: relationship to the AL of mobilizing
- Infancy and childhood—increasing skills
- Adolescence and young adulthood—peak performance
- Later years—decreasing agility and stamina

Dependence/independence in mobilizing
- Increasing independence in childhood, to adulthood
- Dependence on another person
- Body-worn aids } for aided independence
- External aids
- Transport mode—to school, work, shops; for leisure

Factors influencing mobilizing
- Biological
  —adequacy of musculoskeletal and nervous systems
  —body posture/gait
  —muscle strength/mass/tone
  —congenital/hereditary interference with function
  —effects of trauma, disease
- Psychological
  —intelligence level; temperament; values; beliefs; motivation
  —knowledge about benefits of exercise and prevention of injury
  —general attitudes
  —attitudes to dependence and disability
- Sociocultural
  —social class/tradition/religion
  —work activities/transport
  —leisure activities/transport
  —effects of mechanical advances on lifestyle
  —dependence affecting role in relation to family, work, leisure
- Environmental
  —housing conditions and environs
  —local climate and terrain: influence on work/ hobbies
  —effect of energy source on transport of people and goods
- Politicoeconomic
  —community amenities
  —safety of streets/crossings and prevention of injury
  —legal requirements for access to, and mobility in, buildings
  —availability of exercise facilities for leisure

Index

Notes: the abbreviation AL refers to Activities of Living and page numbers in italics refer to information in the Appendices.